The 8 Best Diets of the 21st Century

Maple Grove Press

*Please note: this text contains large excerpts from other works by the same publisher

CONTENTS:

Fad diets come and go like the changing seasons. They go in and out of style. As soon as you think you've found the best one, there's a new one arising that everyone is claiming is the be-all-end-all. What makes matters worse is that medicine can't always agree on the best approaches to dieting and weight loss. There are so many factors involved and so many conflicting opinions — it's enough to make your head spin.

As someone who has struggled with weight for years and has tried many different diets, I've discovered something that most diet-pushers don't want you to know: there is NO magic diet that works wonders for everyone. They all work to some degree and not in other ways. It all depends on what your priorities are and your level of commitment. As many psychologists say, it's better to commit to something and give it your all (even if it's not the 100% solution) than to spend all your time trying to find the perfect solution and thus, not committing to anything.

So many people jump from diet to diet hoping for a quick fix and when they haven't magically transformed, they hop onto the next one believing that the next one will be the real deal. What results? Stagnated progress, lack of motivation, and lack of belief in yourself that you can do it.

There is no cookie cutter diet that is going to transform everyone's lives across the board. Most diets have pros and cons (some are heavier on the pros while some are heavier on the cons). Most of them can help you lose weight and many of them can help you achieve your health and dietary goals, but not all of them are equal and not all of them are equally suited to you.

So how do you choose?

This book seeks to help you make sense of all the conflicting information out there by compiling a list of the 10 Highest rated diets of the 21st Century. Many criteria have been considered when compiling this list including:

- Popularity, consumer satisfaction with the diet
- Consumer success
- Medical Recommendation
- Research and scientific data
- Safety and Easiness of Execution

By reading this book you'll be able to compare and contrast the strengths and weaknesses of each of the diets included in this list and you'll be able to start to think about which one might align with your lifestyle and goals the most.

There are many approaches. Some diets focus solely on what you do and do not eat, whereas other diets are not restrictive about what you eat, but focus on quantities. Some diets focus primarily on eating schedules while others are more intense lifestyle changes that will revolutionize the way you see food.

For each of the 8 Diets that are examined in this book, you will learn:

- What the benefits and risks are that are associated with the diet
- How to follow the diet
- How to get the most out of the diet
- What you can and cannot eat on the diet
- The biological and scientific explanation of the diet (where applicable)
- The philosophy behind the diet (how it was constructed and why it was constructed)

Of course, nothing in this book should be considered medical advice. This book is merely a collection of information that helps you find a good fit for your dietary goals. As always, you should consult with your physician before starting any new diet. Your physician will be able to help you evaluate a particular diet in light of your unique health circumstances and conditions and you'll be able to make an informed decision based off of your physician's recommendations.

1.   The Ketogenic Diet

In a Nutshell: The Keto Diet is extremely low in carbohydrates, high in healthy fats, with a moderate balance of protein. The body normally uses glucose from carbohydrates as its primary energy source, but when we starve the body of carbohydrates, the body enters a state of ketosis where it uses fatty acids for fuel. This typically results in weight loss as well as a whole host of other benefits.

A more in-depth look at the nutrition:

A keto diet is focused on minimizing the intake of carbs. Because of this, the keto diet is sometimes referred to as a low-carb diet or a low-carb, high-fat (LCHF) diet.

Normally, when you consume something that has a high carb content, two things happen within your body. The carbs are broken down into glucose, which is the easiest molecule that the body can use as a source of energy. The body will also produce insulin to help process the glucose.

Since your body uses the glucose as the primary source of energy, your fats have no immediate use and therefore the body stores them. This is what happens when you are on a normal, high-carb diet. However, when you decrease your intake of carbs through the keto diet, your body goes into a state known as ketosis. This is a natural state that the body uses to help us survive when there's low food intake. In this state, the body breaks down fats in the liver to produce ketones, which are then used as a source of energy.

The end goal of keto cleansing is to get your body into this metabolic state. However, instead of using starvation to do this, the keto diet achieves ketosis by depriving the body of carbohydrates. Since the body is highly adaptive, once you overload it with fats and deprive it of carbs, it will switch to using ketones as the primary source of energy.

Since the aim of keto cleansing is to reduce your intake of carbs, you should avoid grains such as rice, cereal, and wheat, sugars such as honey and maple syrup, fruits such as oranges, bananas, and apples and tubers such as potatoes and yams. Instead, you should increase your intake of meats, leafy greens, above ground vegetables, high-fat dairy, avocados and berries, nuts and seeds, low-carb sweeteners and other fats, such as coconut oil, saturated fats, high-fat salad dressing, and so on.

Some of the Main Benefits of the Keto Diet Are:

Weight loss: If you are trying to shed some weight, undergoing keto cleansing is one of the best ways to do it since ketosis burns the stored fat and converts it into energy. Scientific studies have shown that a keto diet has far better weight loss results than low-fat and higher-carb diets.

Anti-inflammation: The human body can derive energy from sugar or fat. While the body uses sugar as the primary source of energy, fat is preferred in the keto diet because it is healthier and cleaner. Converting fat to energy produces fewer secondary free radicals and reactive oxygen species (ROS). By getting removing sugar from your diet, you decrease your chances of developing chronic inflammation.

Decreased risk of cancer: According to research by the University of South Florida, a keto diet can help lower the risk of getting cancer. All the cells in the body typically use glucose as a source of fuel. However, unlike normal body cells, cancerous cells are not metabolically flexible, which means that they cannot switch to using ketones as a source of energy. Once your body starts using ketones as the primary source of energy, the cancerous cells will starve to death.

Increased muscle mass: The structure of ketones is similar to that of branched-chain amino acids, which are essential for building muscle mass. When your body produces ketones, it frees up these amino acids to be used to increase muscle mass. This is why the keto diet is a favorite for athletes.

Increased energy and normalized hunger: Fat is a better and more reliable source of energy for the body. By converting fats to energy, your body feels more energized during the day. Fats are also more satisfying and keep the body in a satiated state for longer. This keeps hunger pangs at bay and makes you feel full and satisfied after eating.

Control blood sugar: By undergoing keto cleansing, you can control your blood sugar levels because you consume fewer carbs for the body to break down into sugars. Studies have shown that a keto diet is an effective way of preventing and managing diabetes.

Lower insulin levels: When you consume carbs, the body breaks them down into sugars, causing a rise in your blood sugar levels. This in turn leads to production of more insulin. If this goes on for some time, you might develop insulin resistance, which can quickly progress to type 2 diabetes if unchecked. By limiting your intake of carbs through keto cleansing, you can reduce your risk of developing type 2 diabetes.

Better mental focus: Many people undergo keto cleansing specifically to increase their mental performance. Ketones are a better source of fuel for the brain compared to glucose. By keeping your carb intake low, you avoid spikes in blood sugar levels. This helps improve your focus and concentration.

Some of the Risks of the Keto Diet:

Most Doctors advise their patients to only strictly adhere to the ketogenic diet for temporary periods of time (2 or 4 week cleanses). A low carbohydrate life style is more sustainable, but a strict keto lifestyle is seen by some experts as dangerous for long term practice.

Some Risks of Long Term Practice of the Keto Diet:

-Some people can lose muscle mass and struggle with fatigue

-some people have had issues with dehydration since they shed so much water weight

-Many people augment their sugar-free diets with chemical filled artificial sweeteners that can be more unhealthy than regular sweeteners.

What to Eat on the Keto Diet:
-Vegetables

-Berries

-Nuts, and natural Nut Butters

-Butter and oils

-Meat, and fish (especially fattier fish like salmon)

-Eggs

-Dairy (cheese, cream, yogurt etc, as long as its natural and in moderation)

What you Should Not Eat:
-Sugars

-Grains

-Pasta, rice, bread etc.

-Carb heavy vegetables: potatoes, corn etc.

-Fruit (with the exception of berries and some melons)

-processed foods and any type of refined sugars

-any type of sweetened drink (both naturally or artificially sweetened

Keto Cooking:

1. **Learn to love veggies:** if you already love veggies, then I'm sure I don't need to convince you. But the number one thing that can help you fall in love with veggies is their versatility. You can do ANYTHING with them. Fry them, steam them, sear them, roast them, bake them, puree them, grill them etc. The best part of keto diet is that most veggies are free reign. Veggies are low in calories and carbs and high in vitamins and nutrients making them the perfect replacement or alternative for carbs in your dishes. If you're in a pinch, or don't have fresh veggies on hand I have a super easy delicious veggie side-dish hack for you.

Super Easy Veggie Fix:

1 bag frozen vegetables (cauliflower, broccoli, California medley etc).

Italian Seasoning

Salt & Pepper

Garlic Powder

Grated Parmesan (the kind in a can is fine)

1 tbsp. butter (optional)

Directions:

Microwave the vegetables according to the package directions with a few tbsp. of water to steam them. When they're done steaming, add the butter (if you decided to use it) then just sprinkle on the rest of the ingredients and stir. The result: a delicious keto-friendly veggie side dish. (I even eat this for my meal if I'm in a hurry).

*The best part is, it takes about 5 minutes of your time, it uses ingredients you probably always have on hand, and it tastes delicious—like something you'd get at a fancy restaurant.

2.   Substitute and improvise: your favorite recipe calls for pasta? Mashed potatoes? Rice? No problem! Just because the recipe is carb heavy doesn't mean you can't tweak it to make it work for your diet. There are always veggie or keto friendly alternatives. Here are a few of my favorites:

- Spaghetti: spaghetti squash
- Noodles: tofu noodles packed in water (ready to eat, you can get at most grocery stores)
- Rice: cauliflower rice
- Potatoes: cauliflower or eggplant
- Mashed potatoes: cauliflower mash
- Bread crumbs: dried grated parmesan cheese
- Pasta: zucchini noodles
- Rice: bean sprouts and/or chopped cabbage sautéed
- Tortillas and wraps: bib lettuce (lettuce wraps) or low carb wraps

The list goes on. There are so many creative ways to make healthy substitutions in your recipes. With the right combination of herbs and spices and the right flavor combinations, you can make anything taste good. And with the recipes in this book, I promise that the flavors are so great you won't even miss the carbs.

3 Count/Keep Track: set a goal for yourself and keep track of it. Whether you want to limit the number of carbs you take in or whether you are focusing on some other metric, keep track of it and try to stick to it. It's very easy to say "I am trying to eat low-carb," but if you don't pay any attention to how many carbs you're actually eating/cooking with you may not be accomplishing anything. There are many foods that people consume a lot of and they have no clue what the nutritional value is.

Set a goal or a threshold for yourself and be meticulous about counting the nutritional values of everything you ingest. When cooking, consider everything that goes into the recipe. At first it will seem like a big pain to tally up the nutrition facts for all ingredients in your recipe, but you will get used to it and start to remember the basic nutritional values of the foods you most often eat and cook with.

The great news for you is that I've already done all that hard work for you in this book. The carbs, calories, protein and fat content are listed at the bottom of every recipe.

4   You don't have to break the bank: many people think keto cooking has to be expensive especially because you are eating more expensive proteins like meat, and cutting out cheap starches like pasta and rice. Just because you're eating keto does not mean you have to spend a lot of money. Meat can be expensive, but it can also be very affordable depending on what kind you buy.

    a.   The great thing about the slow cooker is that it dresses up the meat for you and makes even very cheap cuts of meat taste tender and delicious.

    b.   Pork and chicken are your friends. They're cheap, and easy to work into any recipe.

c. Shop the sales—look at what cuts of meat are on sale at your supermarket on a particular week and plan your meal accordingly.

d. Get your produce from farmer's markets and stands whenever possible. You can get quality produce for amazing prices at these places. Avoid the big box grocery stores and chains for produce. The quality is usually lacking and they're almost always more expensive.

5 **Splurge when it counts:** it can be tempting to fall back on cheap starches and carbs because they are an economical and filling option, but don't fall for it. Consider the long-term consequences: If you make that a habit, you will slip further and further from your dietary goals. Poor physical fitness can lead to poor health which can lead to expensive medical care etc. Just remind yourself that you're saving money in the long run. See it as an investment in yourself so that when you're feeling guilty about splurging on pricier healthy ingredients, remind yourself that it's worth a few more dollars now for a lifetime of benefits and savings in the long run.

6 **Avoid low fat/low cal. ingredients in your cooking:** low fat products/ingredients are deceptive because they seem like a no-strings-attached healthier version of the regular version of that product/ ingredient. However, low fat products are usually loaded with extra sugars and sweeteners to improve the flavor and make up for the reduction in fat and calories. This means that low fat/low cal. versions of ingredients typically have significantly more carbs than their original versions. Stick with whole foods and natural products. Read the labels and compare. Don't just automatically assume something is better for you because it's low cal/low fat. Besides, you need high fat foods to offset the protein you are ingesting and make up for the carbs you are lacking

7   Keto dessert is possible: when you started your keto journey you may have thought you'll never get to satisfy your sweet tooth again. You may have thought you'll never get to have chocolate or eat sweets again, but that's just not the case. You can still have dessert. There is even a small "slow cooker keto dessert" section in this book. With so many sugar-free and low-sugar options available now, low carb dessert has never been more possible.

And you don't always need to make a whole dessert. If you're like me, sometimes you just need a sweet snack to kill that sweet tooth.

- Dark chocolate,
- berries with whipped cream,
- peanut butter
- yogurt with honey or protein powder—

These are just a few of the simple great ways to kill your sweet tooth. And once you try the desserts in this book, you won't even feel like you're dieting.

8   Get some gadgets: invest in a few gadgets that will make your life easier when it comes to keto cooking and it will make your cooking more fun and creative.

Here are a few ideas: (this is by no means an exhaustive list, and you don't need all of these, but consider stocking up on a few).

- **Slow Cooker** (a must for this book)
- **Vegetable Spiraler** (great for making veggie noodles)
- **Vegetable slicer** (very multi-functional, great for veggie pasta)
- **Blender**
- **Standing mixer/hand beaters** (for keto baking)
- **Scale** (weight and measure)

- **Meat thermometer** (get a digital instant-read one if you can)
- **Immersion blender**
- **Grater**
- **Julienne vegetable peeler**

Obviously, there is much more that can be said about the ketogenic diet, and there are tons of studies and conflicting opinions and arguments about the pros and cons and the do's and don'ts. If you listen to them all, you'll drive yourself crazy. Just keep it simple for yourself and focus on one thing at a time and I promise you will make amazing strides towards your goals.

Consensus: if you are very overweight the keto diet may be a great weight loss solution for you in the short term. A low carb lifestyle is more sustainable and healthy for long term practice with periodic strict keto cleanses to help keep the fat off. Do not attempt this diet without first consulting your doctor to see if it's right for you.

2.   The Paleo Diet:

In a nutshell: a primal way of eating. An embracing of our early human roots, the paleo diet is centered around the premise that most of our modern understanding of nutrition is misguided and we have artificially manufactured much of the food we eat, so this lifestyle seeks to go back to basics and eat only naturally occurring foods and foods that would have been available to ancestors during the hunting and gathering phase of civilization.

An In-depth Understanding:

The paleo diet goes by many pseudonyms, including the Stone Age Diet and the caveman diet. There is plenty of truth to these statements. In truth, the paleo diet is short for the Paleolithic diet, but what in the world does this mean? The answer lies in our history. In order for us to understand the paleo diet, we must first gain an understanding and solid appreciation of human history over the past few thousand years. We will skip contentious creationist versus evolutionist accounts and delve into when humans first began interacting with each other.

In the beginning (pun intended), what modern scientists refer to as homo sapiens, lived in small bands and groups, mostly sleeping in trees, and creating rudimentary tools from the rocks they found. These caveman-esque homo sapiens had one really good skill: they could learn. Distinguishing them from other primates was their uncanny ability to pick out what the sharpest tool was, and begin using that as a weapon.

Over time, human beings realized that these sharp rocks could be used for other purposes. The caveman world was one filled with peril – not only did humans have to contend with wild bears, tigers, and other large animals, even smaller ones like wolves could cause serious harm to them. Over a long period of time, wolves would approach humans looking for a new source of food. Sometimes, even against their own will, humans would throw food to the wolves to appease them or so that they would leave them alone. Over generations of this behavior, it soon became apparent that humans could theoretically work with the wolves. These wolves slowly turned into domesticated animals that we now call dogs. Notice how what used to be a predator slowly became not only 'man's best friend' but also ended up working with the human to track down and kill big game—and here is where some food facts come in.

Our caveman ancestors did not farm or mass-produce products as we do today. However, they did one interesting thing: they left the cave. Unlike other primates, our ancestors learned how to use their brains to hunt and gather food, grouping into collectives, and creating tools to better equip themselves. This is the distinguishing factor between humans and other primates.

Here is an interesting example of this divergence in the form of a scientific experiment. Scientists in the 20th century decided to tie a banana from a ceiling place a few monkeys and a chair in the room. The monkeys soon figured out that if they place the chair under the banana, they could climb up the chair and reach their prize. However, if the scientists gave these monkeys a bunch of lumber, some nails, and a hammer, the monkeys would not be able to assemble a chair and use it to reach the banana. Humans have this capability, and it is because of this that we managed to leave the cave, so to speak.

Leaving the cave allowed humans not only infinite possibilities, but also many dangers. Our hunter-gatherer ancestors could really only rely on two food sources: wild game and berries. Two interesting developments occurred. First, our ancestors somehow realized that heating up the meat that they ate made them less sick. And to this day, humans have evolved stomachs that can only digest cooked meat (the fire burns the bacteria and allows us to safely eat meat).

Naturally, our ancestors did not know much about germs or bacteria, but what transpired was that those humans that ate cooked meat ended up not getting sick as often as those who did not. After generations of this, only those humans who consistently ate cooked meat survived, leaving us (their offspring) to be unable to eat uncooked meat without getting sick.

In fact, humans are the only animals that have to eat cooked meat. No other carnivore in the animal kingdom eats their meat cooked. The second development is just as interesting. There are more poisonous mushrooms, berries, legumes, and fish than almost anything else in the world. So how did our ancestors know how to forage for specific ones that are healthy for us? The answer lies in thousands of years of trial and error. Our ancestors realized that some berries are poisonous while others are delicious. Our senses adapted to help us determine the difference—humans are astutely aware of rotting in fruits and vegetables, we can tell if something is rotting not only with our eyes, but also with our senses of smell and taste. These qualities helped humans survive after they left the cave and allowed them to adapt to their environments.

Survival of the fittest then took on a different appearance a few thousand years ago. Leaving the cave was one thing, but humans for thousands of years remained nomadic or semi-nomadic, chasing after wild animals and collecting and hunting berries along the way. This is humanity at its most primitive (and some say, at its healthiest). Hunting and gathering allowed humans to not only gain strength and intelligence, but also to increase in population.

It was during this period—called the Paleolithic Era (sound familiar)—that humans developed into stronger tribes, bands, and chiefdoms. It was also during this time period that we began to incorporate words into our vocabulary. For thousands of years, humans communicated solely using body language and rudimentary noises.

Over time, we developed speech: using words and sounds to express ideas, feelings, and emotions. This speech allowed humans to hunt in a more systematic fashion and remotely. Suddenly, humans could plan ahead, trick animals, and set up traps for their prey. Speech also allowed humans to spread ideas from one tribe to another, meaning that what once was a jagged rock found in the surface could one day turn into a spear. Then a drastic revolution occurred, one that would define the meaning of civilization: our brains got ahead of ourselves, and we began to farm.

There are three qualities needed for a civilization to develop: language, fire, and agriculture. We touched upon the human developments for language and fire; however, it's the third quality that interests the paleo diet. After thousands of years and many iterations of trial and error, humans realized that if they planted the seeds of the fruits they ate in the ground and waited a few months, these new crops could provide more food.

This was true of many foods that humans ate, ranging from cereals such as wheat and barley, to fruits such as grapes and bananas.

Any farmer will tell you that it does not take one year for a harvest, and humans for a long time remained semi-nomadic—farming for a few months and then returning to their hunter-gatherer lifestyles. Over time, this agricultural revolution enticed humans to remain in one spot indefinitely. The word 'revolution' in this sense is not hyperbole. It is precisely because of agriculture that humans have been able to coalesce into civilizations. Because we were able to remain in one location, we began building—and build we did. Roads, cities, permanent buildings, places of worship, homes, and armories began to spring wherever humans lived.

Simultaneous with the agricultural revolution came our increased closeness with livestock. Humans soon learned how to domesticate not only wolves into dogs, but also cattle, sheep, goats, chickens, and even bees. Closer contact with these animals not only allowed for us to tame them, but also spread diseases from animals to humans at a horrifying rate. For many generations, humans died from anthrax, tetanus, and salmonella, all diseases transmitted to them by the animals they worked and lived with.

However, domesticating livestock was not part of the original diet of our ancestors. Chickens, for example, have evolved so resolutely that they now cannot live by themselves. They can only exist because humans care for them—wherever there are chickens, there are humans. Because of farming and taking care of livestock, humans were now able to increase the size of their tribe from a few dozen foresters to thousands upon thousands of people, capable of building the Pyramids and the Great Wall of China. But something changed within us along the way, a change that for most of human history has been considered positive, but has recently led us to unhealthy living conditions: our diet is now based off cereals, grains, sugars, processed oils, and (I know, controversially enough) alcohol.

Enter the paleo diet. The paleo diet seeks to revert modern day humans back to the hunter-gatherer days of yesteryear. Farming may have had positive impacts for our species over the course of the past five thousand years, but in more sedentary lifestyles, it poses significant problems, including propensities for obesity. The paleo diet requires that those eating food must copy the actions of their Paleolithic ancestors. These were our hunter-gatherer forefathers who predominantly ate lean meat, fish, berries, and nuts. The paleo diet also restricts eating food that can be mass-produced in farms and food that we did not eat during our hunter-gatherer days (e.g., chicken). So what foods do paleo dieters eat? Here are the top ten things to know about the paleo diet, along with tips and tricks on how to meal prep the paleo way.

What To Eat

1.   Vegetables

First and foremost, our ancestors ate roots. I know this sounds absolutely disgusting, so let me elaborate before you close this book. All vegetables are roots. Carrots, onions, squash, pumpkins, zucchini, shallots, broccoli, watercress, cauliflower, and yams are all vegetables (aka: roots). They are all also extremely healthy and nutritious. Even though our ancestors had little idea of what vitamins are (clue: vital amino acids), they soon realized that these foods kept them healthy and gave them energy. There is one problem with eating vegetables though. They are mostly water. While water is good for you, it does not feed humans. We need more that just water if we are going to expend the amount of energy that we need to in order to lose weight. This brings us to the next most important facet of the paleo diet: lean meats and fish.

## 2.	Protein

Before the age of agricultural farming and domestication of livestock, humans needed to supplement their diets with proteins. Unlike fats or carbohydrates, proteins are building blocks necessary for muscle growth and repair. Proteins are large biomolecules consisting of long chains of amino acids.

However, not all proteins are created alike, and there are thousands of different types of proteins. The proteins found in bodybuilding supplements are very different from those found in lean meat, fish, and peanuts. The proteins consumed by our hunter-gatherer ancestors were those of wild game, fish, and, in moderation, eggs. Because of this, proteins found in this type of food are encouraged under the paleo diet.

However, other proteins, such as those found in chicken and other white meat poultry are more likely to be discouraged in the paleo diet. While eggs are not taboo per se, eating eggs as a sole source of protein is problematic for the paleo diet, as they are byproducts of domesticated chickens. Rather, it would be better to eat them as supplements to a much larger protein diet. Along the same vein, while eating lean meat is encouraged, drinking copious amounts of milk is not, precisely because of the domesticated nature of the cow, which is a development that occurred during the agricultural revolution and did not exist during the Paleolithic Era.

3.   Fruits

The next food item common in the paleo diet is fruits. Even though most are farmed, their genetic makeup has not changed much. But, just like proteins, we need to make sure that we are eating the right kinds of fruits. Citrus fruits occupy the lion's share of attention for paleo dieters—they possess the right kinds of amino acids, vitamins, and fiber. For example, paleo dieters often single out grapefruits as the single most nutritious fruits in the market. They are loaded with Vitamin C (around 20% of your daily dose of the vitamin), they help lower cholesterol, and contain almost as much citric acid as lemons but without the bitterly sour taste.

The paleo diet also encourages consuming grapes, kiwi, melons, apples, and so on. However, there are fruits loaded with starch that the paleo diet treats with caution. Bananas, for example, are one of the starchier fruits dominant in our diet. The difference between starches and other carbohydrates is that starches consist of large amounts of glucose in the carbohydrate chain. Normal carbohydrates (also colloquially known as carbs) simply consist of carbon, hydrogen, and oxygen atoms, hence the name.

The difference between regular carbohydrates and starches is that, when broken down, starches possess a lot more sugar molecules. Sugar, for what it's worth, is made up of a carbon ring surrounded by hydrogen and oxygen atoms. While bananas are the fruits with the most amount of starches, there are also many starchy vegetables that the paleo diet tends to avoid. A solid example of one of these vegetables is the potato. As for fruits that the paleo diet suggests, generally seasonal fruits are the way to go. However, in modern day society, it is not as necessary to abide by this rule, though it can be encouraged. In any case, seasonal fruit is generally cheaper to buy than non-seasonal fruit in your local supermarket.

4.   Nuts & Seeds

Nuts and seeds are also important components of the paleo diet. These little miracles have astounding percentages of valuable fats, oils, proteins, and vitamins. Cashews, walnuts, sunflower seeds, and almonds are jam packed with nutritious vitamins and fatty acids needed for the paleo diet. These are what our hunter-gatherer ancestors were largely after. They realized that these seeds and nuts carried with them large amounts of necessary proteins and fats that not only helped keep them alive, but also were easily stored and kept for long winters.

Unlike many other foods, nuts and seeds, by nature, are designed to remain fresh for longer periods of time than meat, fruits, and vegetables. Additionally, because they are small and lightweight, they could be carried from place to place as our ancestors chased after wild animals. Currently, we can keep them in lunchboxes on our way to work.

5. Condiments

Finally, the paleo diet is acutely aware of what we cook with. Generally, humans have churned cream enough to make butter, added salt, and cooked with that product. Butter, however, is largely a byproduct of domesticated cows. Luckily, there are plenty of other ingredients that we can cook with that do not include butter. Olive oil is probably the easiest ingredient to cook with and is much healthier for us than butter.

Not only is it rich in unsaturated fats (the good type – the bad type is saturated fat), it is also plentiful and tasty. Other oils are just as good for cooking, but not nearly as universal as olive oil. Coconut oil, walnut oil, and macadamia nut oil are also extremely nutritious and taste great. Where these oils hit hard though, is the bank. They are generally more expensive and rarer than olive oil. However, unlike olive oil, they are less likely to be adulterated by other chemicals.

One of the unfortunate byproducts of the Industrial Age has been the human propensity for adulterating their food products, ranging from injecting corn syrup into honey to mixing extra virgin olive oil with additives. There are a few oils that we should be wary of: vegetable oils and palm oils. While they look (and sometimes taste) similar to olive oil, they are nowhere near the same thing. These oils tend to be largely refined, meaning that the original nutrients inherent in their nature have been burned away to produce a condensate that is not as healthy as before.

The problem is, because they are plentiful and cheap, we tend to cook with them. Nonetheless, if shopping wisely, we can use olive oils for our paleo diets to make healthy and cost-effective meals without having to resort to these unhealthy oils filled with saturated fat that clogs our arteries.

What Not To Eat

1.   **Cereals & Grains**

We have touched upon what paleo dieters do not eat, but let's expand on these a bit. The main difference between the paleo diet and the modern diet that most Americans abide by is the consumption of cereals and grains. Human mass consumption of cereals and grains became prevalent during the agricultural revolution, when we began harvesting wheat, rice, buckwheat, quinoa, oats, rye, barley, and even corn. Cereals are essentially a type of grass that humans consume. We realized that we can plant this grass and have huge pastures of it for our growing populations.

In reality, cereals are the primary reason why we can feed seven billion people in this world. Similar to nuts and seeds, they are easily stored in granaries, can be dried and eaten months later, and stop hunger. In this sense they are good. However, if we are struggling with obesity, consuming more and more cereals is only going to exacerbate the problem. They are great for keeping us alive in times of famine, but not for keeping us healthy. Even though we may not see it, we are consuming more cereals than we think.

2.   **Corn**

Ever traveled through the center of the United States and thought, "man, those are a lot of cornfields?" Subconsciously, you might be thinking that the average person does not eat all that much corn. Most of us eat corn once a month or during the holidays. So why is so much of it being produced?

There are a few answers. Some of it is being produced for ethanol, and is therefore inedible. Some of it is being exported, and some of it is being used to feed livestock. However, much of the corn that is produced in the United States is converted to corn syrup. This is one of sugar's main aliases. Corn syrup is made of starch and is found in almost every processed food, which brings us to the next item that the paleo diet (along with many others) discourages: processed food.

3.   Processed Foods

Here's a neat rule of thumb: if a third grader cannot pronounce what you are eating, then do not eat it. Processed foods include all prepackaged snacks, sodas, and all frozen food. Essentially, any food that is pre-packaged is considered processed food. You can normally distinguish between processed foods and healthy ones by the ingredients. Xanthan gum, monosodium glutamate, hydroxybenzoate do not exist in the wild, and are not part of the paleo diet.

Here's another rule of thumb: when shopping in the supermarket, processed foods are generally in the middle section, while vegetables, dairy, meat, and fruits are around the edges. If you want to shop like a paleo dieter, generally speaking, avoid the middle of the supermarket. That's where the processed food is (you can also tell because it has a longer shelf life). Any food that has a shelf life of over one month can be guaranteed to be not part of the paleo diet.

4.   Alcohol

The next non-paleo ingredient is alcohol. Now before you close this book in anger, there are a few exceptions (exhale). Most alcohol consumed in the United States is beer, which is largely made up of hops, barley, grains, and malt. None of these ingredients are actually good for you—at the very least, they are not bad for you if you consume them in little to moderate quantities.

Other alcohols, such as vodka, are produced from fermented potatoes, which are not paleo. The same is true of sake, which is made of rice, and rum, which is a sugar-based product. Whiskey is largely composed of rye or barley, and sometimes mixed with wheat. While these types of alcohols are not heavy in these grains, they do contain them.

One pint of beer, for its part, is equivalent to eating seven slices of bread in terms of the grains that are included in this beverage. This is less extreme for whiskey or vodka. There is one alcohol, however, that meats most of the paleo requirements, and that is wine. Distilled from grapes, wine is made of fruits, and having one glass of wine with dinner is acceptable for the paleo diet. Be careful, however, as out of all the alcoholic beverages that were mentioned, wine is the one with the most calories. That means that consuming more than one glass of wine per meal may increase your caloric intake much more than you possibly think.

5.   Too Much Salt & Sugar

Finally, unnecessary salts and sugars are not part of the paleo diet. While it is tempting to cook with extra salt to enhance the flavor of many foods, remember that acids also increase their flavor, meaning that when you think that you need to use more salt in your food, you may be able to squeeze some lemon juice into your dish.

Salt is an interesting food choice for us. Our paleo ancestors did not necessarily use salt to cook—they used it to store meats and fish. Before refrigeration, the best way to store sliced meats was to salt them. Because salt dehydrates, these meats would harden and were able to be preserved throughout the winter. Only later did we begin using salt for cooking, realizing that it enhances the flavor of whatever it is that we are eating.

Another interesting factoid about salt is that it's poisonous. You may not think that this is true because we all consume salt. However, our tongues have evolved to detect salt in very small quantities because if we eat too much of it, we dehydrate ourselves. For dieting purposes, another reason to avoid salt is that it makes us look slightly fatter. Again, because salt dehydrates us (and we are around 70 percent water), salt ends up making us drink more fluids and making us feel more bloated.

Ever wondered why you look a bit skinnier in the morning than at night? It's because your body has flushed out a lot of the salt from your system, meaning that you need less water. On the other hand, after consuming salt in three meals during the day, you soon realize that you've put that (water) weight back on. An easy fix for dieters is to limit sodium (salt) intake, especially during breakfast.

Sugarcane sugar is not necessarily bad for you, but to consume it in excess is unhealthy. Vogue new diets include honey and agave nectar as substitutes for sugar, but in reality, your body digests and processes these sugars in a similar way that it processes sugarcane sugar. The main difference between these products and what we think of when we envision sugar is the degree to which it is processed. The more processed a sugar is, the more sweet elements are extracted and the less healthy it is for your body. These sugars and their derivatives are also found in most processed foods, which according to the paleo diet, should also be avoided.

Basics:

How your diet will change by Following the Paleo Diet:

-increase intake of protein

-Obtain most of your daily carbohydrate intake from non-starchy fruits and vegetables

-increase fiber intake

-preference of unsaturated and monounsaturated fats instead of saturated fats

-increased intake of vitamins and minerals

Benefits:

-you are virtually eliminating all processed and unnatural foods so you rid your body of harmful chemicals and additives that have been linked to all sorts of cancers and diseases, plus you boost your intake of antioxidants, vitamins and minerals naturally through the healthy foods you consume

-by eliminating processed foods and sugars, you will be able to lose weight and maintain a healthy weight once you've reached your desired weight.

-Many studies have shown that the paleo diet improves "gut health" helping you better process and digest the food you eat contributing to better absorption of the nutritive elements of your food, plus it will make you feel better and more "regular" with your digestion."

-no focus on calorie counting. In some ways, it's very simple. You just follow the guidelines for what to eat and what not to eat, and the rest is up to you.

-there is a very active paleo "community" both online and in real life. You'll find it easy to find a plethora of information, recipes, and support for your lifestyle.

Risks:

While there aren't many risks, per say, there are some things to consider:

-it can be difficult to maintain since it is a rather restrictive diet. To follow it strictly, you need to be very committed and have a lot of self-control

-always buying paleo substitutes and special ingredients can get quite expensive

-depending on your activity level, you may find you have less energy because of the decrease in carb intake

Consensus: this is a relatively risk-free diet that can be great for both weight-loss and maintenance if you have the self-control for it. If you're interested in living a more "natural" life and are inspired by the embracing of your prehistoric roots, perhaps the paleo diet is for you.

3. The Mediterranean Diet:

In a nutshell: as the name suggests, this is a way of eating that comes from the regions surrounding the Mediterranean Sea that focuses on natural eating without restricting food groups, with a consumption of healthy fats and an elimination of processed foods, hydrogenated fats, and refined sugars.

Hailed By Many as "The World's Healthiest Diet: People in the Mediterranean region have been eating this way for centuries and have been enjoying the wonderful health benefits almost unintentionally. That's the joy of this lifestyle—it's almost effortless. You don't have the unnatural side effects, chemical imbalances or hunger that you experience when following other diet regimens because this lifestyle focuses on adding nutrients to your diet instead of taking them away.

Less of a diet and more of a lifestyle, the Mediterranean way of eating focuses on enriching your diet with fruits and vegetables, grains, beans, and fish foods that have been linked to a whole host of amazing health benefits. The Mediterranean diet is regularly praised by scientists as one of the healthiest diets of all time.

Amazing Benefits of the Mediterranean Diet:

There are many reasons why someone might decide to implement the Mediterranean Diet into their life, and weight loss is only the beginning. While it is true, that you can experience amazing weight loss benefits from following the Mediterranean diet there are many other benefits you may not be aware of.

- **Natural Weight Loss:** Weight loss, but the Natural Way: you are not starving yourself on this diet nor will you find yourself hungry all the time as you would on most other diets. You are not depriving yourself of necessary nutrients the way other diets do sometimes. One of the big differentiators here is the consumption of "healthy fats." This is what leaves you feeling full and satiated without having a negative impact on your health or weight.

- **Nutrient Rich Food:** An increase in probiotics, quality proteins, vitamins, omega-threes and other healthy nutrients and minerals that can be deficient in other diets.

- **Heart Health**: some people may even be "prescribed" this diet by their doctor for the amazing heart-health benefits. Some studies have found that this healthy consumption of mono-unsaturated fats and increase in good cholesterol, plus the increase in omega-threes have been found to likely decrease cardiac death rates by up to 45%

- **Diabetes Prevention And Cure:** Roughly 10% of Americans struggle with diabetes. This is an astounding figure especially when comparing to the stats of people living in the Mediterranean countries. The Mediterranean diet has long been seen as a natural cure for certain types of diabetes because it is naturally low in sugar—and almost completely devoid of processed sugar, and high in fresh fruits and vegetables as well as healthy fats.

- **Cancer Prevention:** The high concentration of health fatty acids, as well as antioxidants and fiber have led many to see a link between the Mediterranean diet and cancer prevention. Plus, this diet is completely devoid of processed foods which are often filled with chemicals that have been linked to cancerous growth.

- **Anti-Aging:** Some studies have shown decreased muscle deterioration in the elderly by up to 60%. Also, there have been many studies linking this type of diet with Alzheimer's and dementia prevention making the Mediterranean diet one of the best diets for anti-aging.

Adoption of this diet in regions outside of the Mediterranean started after a post World War II study on world diets conducted by a team of scientists. Actually, the residents of Crete ranked as the number 1 healthiest group in the study. There are many books that give extensive histories of the Mediterranean diet including many facts and figures showing scientific findings and ranking the benefits of this diet in comparison to others, but as I said, the main purpose of this diet isn't to define it, but rather to help you achieve success once you've made the decision to adopt this lifestyle.

These are just a few of the many, many benefits of this diet. Plus, you as we have already said, this is more than a diet. This is a lifestyle. With this way of eating, you also are invited to adopt the Mediterranean approach to relaxation and recreation. Through the fuel and vitality you will derive from the food you are consuming you will have energy to live a an active lifestyle. Plus you many of these foods can cause a release of endorphins that will improve your mood and alleviate some of your stress allowing you to enjoy life more and not get as caught up In the details.

Indeed, a diet that encourages you to unwind with a glass of dry red wine at night can't be so bad.

What to Eat and What to Avoid:
So what can you eat on the Mediterranean Diet? And What should you Avoid?

This is a diet of balance and moderation so there are very few types of foods that are absolutely forbidden. At most there are foods you should consume moderately or sparingly.

What you should eat a lot of:
- Fruits and veggies: almost all fruits and vegetables are fair game—so mix it up. The great thing about fruits and vegetables is that they're all so vertastile and can be prepared in so many delicious and exciting ways that you'll never get bored.
    - Examples: broccoli, cauliflower, root vegetables (carrots, onions), greens (romaine, kale, spinach), tomatoes, eggplant, zucchini, cucumber, avocados, etc
    - Berries, apples, banans, melons etc. (also dried fruits: dates, raisins, cranberries, cherries etc).
- Nuts: loaded with monounsaturated fats, they will leave you feeling satiated and full—with healthy fat.

o   Example: walnuts, almonds, hazelnuts, cashews, pumpkin seeds etc.

- Beans/Legumes: you will notice many of the recipes here include some form of legumes. Apart from introducing a lot of healthy fiber and protein, they will also help you feel full and stay full.

  o   Garbanzo beans, white beans, black beans, lentils peas etc.

- Grains: any type of whole grain that is unadulterated and unrefined: oats, brown rice, whole wheat, quinoa, couscous etc.

- Fish: high in omega 3's as well as many other nutrients, most americans do not consume nearly enough fish. This is a huge part of the Mediterranean diet:

  o   Trout, tuna, shrimp, shellfish, salmon etc.

- Lean Meats: the better quality the better for you. Grass fed, organic lean beef chicken and pork are very welcome in the Mediterranean diet.

- Eggs and yogurt are great sources of protein and probiotics.

- Go crazy with herbs and spices, not only can they really enhance the flavor of your food, but they can enhance your health too (limit salt intake).

Generally, you'll want to avoid all processed sugars. Natural sugars like fruit are great, but keep the processed sugars to a minimum for best results.

Buy the best quality fruit you can find, and use it as a dessert replacement. If the fruit is actually good quality, you will get used to this new natural sweetness and it will instantly kill your sweet tooth.

7 Steps for Success in the Mediterranean Diet:

1). Olive Oil: you'll notice almost all of these recipes include olive oil. In moderation, olive oil has been shown to increase the good kind of cholesterol and it doesn't cause the negative health effects of processed oils and hydrogenated oils. In moderation, olive oil should be your monounsaturated fat of choice.

*make sure to buy extra virgin olive oil, and I recommend you invest in good quality olive oil not only for flavor, but chances are better that the vital nutrients are preserved in more authentic unprocessed olive oils.

2). No Grain No Gain: some diets instruct you to stay as far away from carbohydrates as possible. While we feel the same about processed and refined carbohydrates, whole grains are essential to the Mediterranean diet Avoid any type of "white" carbs (white bread, white rice, white pasta, white flour) as most of these types of carbs have been bleached and are now devoid of any beneficial nutrients and often contain harmful chemicals.

With wholegrains, you are consuming mostly unprocessed carbohydrates with their nutrients still intact. You will get the filling and satiating feeling from consuming carbohydrates while still benefitting from the nutrients.

3). A glass of wine a day keeps the doctor away:

For heart health, dry red wine in moderation is not only acceptable but encouraged in the Mediterranean diet. Places like Italy and Greece just wouldn't be the same if you had to give up wine, so let's be thankful for that. Limit yourself to a glass or half a glass per day. It's great way to unwind before bed.

4). Fish are friends, also food: as stated previously, most Americans do not eat enough fish. Apart from being a great source of quality protein with low levels of fat, most fish provide you with a healthy dose of omega-3 fatty acids (the good kind). Shop the sales, and don't be afraid to splurge a little for Salmon and Trout on occasion. See it as an investment in your health and treat yourself.

5). Lean red meat in moderation: Fatty red meat should be the exception and not the rule in the Mediterranean Diet. Leaner red meats especially lamb are fine in moderation, but fatty meats like beef ribs and steaks and burgers should be reserved for special occasions and otherwise avoided. But once you try a chargrilled salmon burger, or tuna steaks, you'll forget all about your burger.

6). Beans are Best: lentils, cannellini beans, garbanzo beans etc. are all very important to this diet. Try to get daily portions of legumes. I even like black beans or stewed lentils on my eggs in the morning. Not only are they a great source of fiber and protein, but they're low in fat, so you still feel very nice and full without loading up on fat.

7). Pair the diet with an active lifestyle: eating health is just one piece of the health puzzle (albeit one of the most important pieces). And since you'll be saving so much time by prepping your meals (with this book), you should have even more free time to pursue active leisure. The Mediterranean way isn't so much sweating buckets in the gym, but walking on a summer's night at sunset, or playing tennis with friends, or hiking in the foothills or riding a bike. Whatever your "active leisure" choose something you actually enjoy. Very few of us enjoy going to the gym, so choose something you'll actually look forward to doing in your free time. That way, you'll actually do it.

Risks of the Mediterranean Diet:

-there really are very few (if any risks) but some experts say this diet is too low in calcium so you may actively need to watch your calcium intake and boost wherever possible for bone health

-some people may find weight loss to be too slow or stagnant with this diet (typically the reason is because they're consuming too much fat)

Consensus:

If you're more concerned about overall health and well-being and less concerned about rapid weight-loss, this diet may be for you. It's not that restrictive and allows for a varied and well-balanced diet. For most people it's better for maintaining a healthy weight than rapidly losing weight. If you're more of an olive oil person than a butter person and more of a red wine person than a beer person, this diet is for you.

4. Intermittent Fasting:

In a nutshell: this diet isn't concerned with what you eat, it's only concerned with when you eat (and to some degree how much). By limiting the window of time where you eat every day, you cut out a significant amount of calories which typically results in weight loss.

The term literally means occasional fasting, or not eating, during a given period. Broadly, there are two main forms of intermittent fasting. The first of these involves occasional days off from eating. At the more severe end, which would consist of a one-day-eating, one-day-not regime to the more common kind of routine where there is normal eating for six days of the week, and then one day not eating. This type of fasting would reduce calorie intake by over 14 per cent.

A little clarification here. If we decided to fast on Tuesdays, so our last meal was, say, seven pm on Monday evening, and our next would be breakfast on Wednesday morning, at say seven am, then our fast would actually be of 36 hours, which is a long period under normal circumstances.

Therefore, usually, a twenty-four hour fast would consist of the final meal on the Monday, with the next meal being dinner on the Tuesday, which would represent a full twenty-four hours. Various developments from 24-hour fasts have come about, probably the best known being the 5:2 diet. We will look at this in more detail later, but briefly this involves a week split into five days of normal eating, with two days of much reduced calories, for example down to just 500 on these days.

The second form of intermittent fasting is often called time restricted fasting, or TRF. In this, eating is limited to certain hours of the day. A 16:8 mix is often used where a 16 hour fast is combined with an eight-hour period in which meals can be taken. Unfortunately, for the epicures among our readers, that doesn't mean that there can be an eight-hour binge, but in practice it means that a meal is consumed at the beginning and end of the period, usually lunch and dinner.

Of course, this does mean that the commonly held truism that breakfast is the most important meal of the day is challenged, since it is usually breakfast that is lost. However, as we will see later, the theory that we cannot manage without breakfast is one that does not have quite the scientific backing as might be claimed by our elders.

What is actually consumed during the fasting periods is open to discussion. Some say just water (it is very important to remain hydrated). Others will allow beverages such as tea and coffee while, as we see above, some views exist that fasting can be taken to mean drastically reducing our calorie intake, but still eating a little.

The Biology:

One of the first biological changes to occur is that blood pressure drops, by about ten percent. This has obvious positive health impacts, although research suggests at the moment that the pressure returns to its previous state when the fasting stops.

Another impact is more mysterious. A characteristic of blood, called – vaguely – an 'embryonic like substance' –

increases. Scientists are still unsure exactly what function this part of our blood performs. There is more evidence of this substance in animals, where it is believed to be a way the body repairs itself from disease. If the same function applies in humans, then the increase in this can only be a positive thing. It will enable blood cells to allow regeneration in the body.

One of the main chemical changes in the body we find from fasting is an increase in a chemical inhibitor, the interestingly named IGFBP-1. Broadly, this is the inhibitor which keeps the aging process stable and free from disease. Clearly, such a benefit is going to help us as we get older.

The part of us inhibited by IGFBP-1 is something we certainly want to be kept in check. IGF-1 is a chemical in our blood linked with the onset of many cancers, and other negatives we experience as we get older. Therefore, the conclusion is that intermittent fasting will protect us from many diseases.

Another change in the body is a reduction in the 'addiction' chemicals the brain produces. It seems as though dopamine, the chemical which gives a feeling of satisfaction, is repressed to some extent, which could have a benefit for addictions, such as certain foods, and even alcohol and nicotine.

As with other areas in this field, research is currently limited, and therefore conclusions are far from certain. However, glutamate and GABA, the chemicals which transfer messages to the brain, may be affected, reducing the crave impact of endorphins. In contrast, other scientists, such as consultant psychiatrist Dr Jonathon Chick, are less sure, feeling that personality probably plays a bigger part in addiction.

It must be remembered that the research is still in its early stages with regards to the internal workings of the body, and therefore the conclusions regarding the impact of intermittent fasting are not certain, but the evidence is growing that it really helps us to stay healthy and free from many of the worst diseases to which mankind is exposed – not only in the present but as we get older as well.

Methods:

The Five:Two Method

The principle behind this approach is that we eat normally for five days of the week and choose two (non-consecutive) days to eat a much-reduced calorie intake. One of the great advantages of this method is the flexibility it offers.

We can pick which two days we like to fast. For example, many people might want to keep their weekends normal, and might sense that their energy levels begin to drop after a week at work. So fasting days of Monday and Wednesday could work very well for them.

The best idea on the fasting days is to aim for two very light meals, perhaps two meals of 300 calories for men, 250 for women. To give an idea, a breakfast of 300 calories looks a bit like a whole wheat English muffin, topped with low fat butter, a small hard-boiled egg, a handful of fruits and a small glass of fruit juice, plus as much water as you want.

A baked potato with sour cream and a water melon side would make a decent dinner at this number of calories, as would a small chicken breast, grilled and served with some green beans and a small side salad.

Lunch could be a bowl of soup with some saltine crackers, or a roasted vegetable salad with a sweet potato, some greens, pepper and eggplant and a light honey dressing. While these are not huge meals, unsurprisingly at their calorie limits, they are still things we might eat anyway for a meal.

On the remaining five days of the week we eat normally, three well balanced meals and a snack. In fact, the portions could be a little bigger if we want, especially for meals following a fasting day. As long as the overall weekly calorie intake is lower than normal, the fast will have the effects we seek.

At the time of writing, there have been no specific studies into the 5:2 diet, but we do know that this is a form of intermittent dieting, and that in itself has some research and lots of anecdotal evidence into its benefits.

The 5:2 diet is a great introduction to intermittent fasting. It is a lot less severe than, say the alternate day method, and is therefore quite easy to get into.

The 16:8 Approach

If the 5:2 approach to intermittent fasting is an easy way to get involved in the program, then the 16:8 version is at least as straightforward. Two nice sized meals are eaten every day, and the body very quickly gets used to the fasting part of the day, particularly as it usually includes eight hours of sleep. In fact, some proponents argue that the eating time can be extended from eight to ten hours. On this basis, there are only six hours of waking time per day when you cannot eat.

Many experts in the field believe that it is after around sixteen hours that most people's bodies enter the 'fasting state'. There does seem, though, to be a slight difference between the genders, with women needing around 14-15 hours to reach their optimum fasting state, men slightly longer.

Leangains was made popular by the fitness expert, Martin Berkhan, in the mid '90's. It really is a no-pain way to improve health and lose weight. First, the fasting state is not especially onerous. Most people will follow the program below, but so long as the fasting period is continuous, it can be adapted to best fit an individual's lifestyle.

Let us start with the evening meal. For most people, this is going to be between 7.00 and 8.00pm. We can say for the purposes of this example that we finish eating at 8.00pm. We then relax and go to bed at, say 11.00pm. A good night's sleep and we are up at 7.00am. Our body will soon get used to not having breakfast, and as we saw earlier, the old adage that breakfast is the most important meal of the day does not have much in the way of science to back it up.

In fact, lots of us already skip this meal, although often not for dietary reasons but because we cannot get ourselves together in the morning. We are the people who then overdo it with other meals – if we could get those under control, our bodies would really experience the benefits. And, we can all reassure ourselves that lunch is not far away.

But there is a plus: with the 16:8 diet: it is fine to have a tea or coffee (even with a splash of milk) in that intervening period. A good cup of Americano (try it black, if you don't already have it that way. The taste is soon acquired, and you will wonder why you ever added milk.), or a green tea will see any lingering pangs of hunger firmly in the background as we make our way through morning, head clear and able to work at pace.

A good lunch, we can have a bigger one than normal if we need it, will keep us going through to dinner in the evening. But, if your body tells you so, as we are not in our fasting period, then a late afternoon snack can keep us buzzing until the main meal of the day.

We have said it often, but it bears repeating. The meals in our non-fasting period can be a little bigger than normal, especially as our body is acclimating to its new regime, but they do still need to be healthy and in moderation. Not small, but remember our aim is to reduce our overall calorie intake. The odd take-away is fine, but a week of curries, Chinese take-away, take out pizzas and a giant spread of Mexican food will be as harmful to us during our intermittent fasting as it would be to anybody not taking part in any healthy eating program.

The fun part of the 16:18 diet is that you can experiment. See how your metabolism handles the change in eating habits. For some, if they confine their eating to an 8 hour window, and fast the remaining 16 hrs (including 8 hrs of sleep), they can basically eat as much as they want during those 8 hrs.

If you train yourself to simply eat until you are full (instead of overeating), you will often find it difficult to consume "too many" calories in your 8 hr window where you're allowed to eat. The secret is training your body to not "over-eat" during these periods.

By the way, one caveat to the above statement is: sugar. Consuming a lot of sugar will almost always cause you to surpass your calorie limit for the day. Natural sugars like fruit, or healthy sugars like organic dark chocolate are fine in moderation, but highly processed sugars, and sugary drinks are not your friend.

If you can manage to eat 2 big healthy filling meals a day with lots of fresh veggies and healthy fats, you will be amazed at how easy it is to shave up to 500 or 600 calories off of every single day. As this compounds and adds up, the pounds will be flying off of you.

Say if you eat a nice big lunch with avocado and cashews and some nice healthy fats that will make you feel full and satisfied. You are going to be full for quite a while. Maybe you eat a light snack at midafternoon, and then a late dinner. You won't need to consume 2500 calories--or 2000 or whatever your daily intake is--in that period of time.

Whether to choose the 5:2 or 16:8 intermittent fasting approach is very much down to the individual. 16:8, or Leangains (because it increases your lean body mass) requires the regular discipline of not eating during the 15-16 hour fast. We will get used to it very quickly, but this is a regular, daily program. Some people become bored with this approach and will begin to break it. For others, who like to plan their days in detail, then it is a perfect method to achieve weight loss.

If the diet of our choice is the 5:2 method, then we need to be the kind of person who is not going to spend our five normal days dreading the 'fasting' days. Again, remember that the word fast is an exaggeration here, on the two days we can still eat. Just not a big amount. However, if we are the kind of person who likes a bit of variety, and who would rather tough it out for 2 days instead of lightly holding back every day, then this route might be the best one for us.

Benefits:

- You will almost certainly lose weight.
- Fasting provides a body cleansing service, which can eliminate poisons from the body. (which will make you feel better, reduce bloating, and reduce your risk of many different types of diseases)

- Because the fasting is reasonable regular, those poisons are less likely to build up.
- It is a cheap way of losing weight and becoming healthier.
- It is an easy way of achieving the above, with no measuring out food or counting calories.
- There are health benefits beyond weight loss. Evidence suggests a number of conditions will be eased by intermittent fasting, and it can delay the onset of others.

- There is evidence that this kind of fasting can actually extend our lifespan.
- There are many types of intermittent fasting, which means that we can select one that best fits our lifestyle and personality.
- You can eat what you want to eat, which makes it easier to keep up.
- Evidence suggests that our bodies adapt very quickly to this kind of fasting, which makes it easier to keep up. We all know the problem of other kinds of diet, where we can crave foods we are not allowed to eat.
- Our overall calorie intake will go down.
- Some evidence suggests that it can increase concentration and mental focus, making our work better.
- Because we feel healthy, our moods are more consistent and better, improving personal relationships.
- The diet is compatible with exercise programss
- Fasting can be a short-term fix, or a long-term lifestyle choice. Both methods will provide some benefit.
- Fasting has, for many years, formed a part of the culture of various societies.

Risks:

- some people had issues with their cortisol levels being too high (stress hormone)
- some people may have issues with energy while the adjust to the diet
- some people have taken the lifestyle to an unhealthy extreme and made it into an eating disorder.
- Do not attempt this diet without first consulting your physician to ensure this is right for you, and closely follow his recommendation for how you

should implement intermittent fasting into your life.

Consensus: if you find other diets too complicated or restrictive and you just want to be able to eat what you want, this diet may be for you. If you have the willpower to actually follow the schedule and not over-binge or eat super calorie dense foods during your eating periods, you may achieve great success with this diet.

5. The Low-Calorie Diet (Calorie Counting):

In a Nutshell: The basic concept of this diet is relatively simple. You lose weight by simply depriving your body of calories. Generally, this is accomplished by consuming fewer calories than you burn in a day. This is primarily a weight-loss centered diet and apart from the whole host of health risks you avoid by being a healthy weight, there aren't a lot of other major reasons people choose this diet other than weight loss.

This diet can be very practical if you like something simple and measurable. Apart from counting calories, there's really nothing else you need to keep track of.

Doing the Math:

One pound of fat is 3500 calories. So, in order to lose a pound of fat, you need to consume 3500 calories less than you've burned. If your goal was to lose 1 pound per week, you would have to eat 500 calories less than you burn each day. To lose ½ pound every week, you'd have to eat 250 fewer calories than you burn every day that week. Pretty simple, right?

But where it gets complicated, is figuring out how many calories you really do burn in one day. Everyone's metabolism is different and of course it also depends on your activity level. For example, someone that has a manual labor job where they're required to move a lot and lift a lot will burn a lot more calories in a day than someone at a desk job. For women, it's different than men, and it also depends on your age and health conditions, medications etc. These are all things that need to be considered. For a very accurate report, you'll want to consult with your physician and after looking at all these questions, they'll be able to pinpoint an estimated number of calories you burn every day. That will allow you to plan how you will go about cutting calories to lose weight.

However, there are simple ways for you to calculate for yourself the range of calories you need each day to maintain your weight. This basically means that if you eat X number of calories each day, you'll neither gain nor lose weight. If you eat fewer calories, you'll start to lose weight, if you eat more calories, you'll start to gain weight.

One pretty simple way of calculating your magic number of calories is simply by experimenting. Eat how you normally would for two weeks keeping close track of how many calories you eat, but not trying to cut calories. Weigh yourself every day and do the math. If you neither gained weight nor lost weight, you're at your magic number of calories. If you gained weight, you'll want to calculate how much and then do the math.

For example: if Sally eats an average of 2100 calories per day, and she weighs herself every morning and she stays roughly the same over the course of two weeks (weight can fluctuate, but you'll notice if you really start gaining or losing), then that means that 2100 calories per day is the amount Sally needs to maintain her weight. Thus, if sally wanted to lose ½ pound every week, she'd need to drop down to 1850 calories per day.

If Sally consumes an average of 2100 calories a day for 2 weeks and at the end of it, she's gained weight, then we know she's already eating too many calories even for weight maintenance.

If at the beginning of the two weeks, Sally weighed 165 pounds, and at the end of the two weeks she weighs 166 pounds, that means she gained 1 pound by eating 2100 calories a day. Thus, to simply maintain her weight, she'd need to consume 1850 calories. To lose weight, she would need to consume even less. For example, if she wanted to lose ½ pound every week, she'd have to consume 1500 calories.

As you can see, this can get quite tricky and its certainly not an exact science. Indeed, it could take weeks of experimenting to find your magic number. However, there are many online tools that aggregate data from all kinds of people and give you a pretty realistic range of numbers to go by.

All you have to do is plug in your current weight, gender and age, and it will tell you how many calories per day you need to consume to maintain your weight. Other more sophisticated services will also ask how active you are and offset the numbers according to your activity level. While that's better than not taking activity into account, it's kind of a vague question that people aren't very good at answering. It's difficult to say how active someone is—and it also depends on their profession and honestly, things just vary from day to day so it can be difficult.

Don't agonize too much over these questions—everything we're dealing with here is going to be estimations for the most part.

Just like finding your target number of calories per day can be a bit imprecise, it can also be difficult to accurately calculate how many calories you actually did consume in a day. Eating out in restaurants complicates this the most. Unless you know every ingredient, the dish is made with, you won't know for sure what the calorie content is. You can make an educated guess and rely on online data that gives you averages of what the calorie content is of typical meals like yours, but unless the restaurant provides nutrition information (and some do), you won't be able to know really how many calories you're consuming.

Also, when cooking for themselves, many people end up forgetting to calculate things like oil if they're sautéing something. The other problem is they just estimate the number of calories in what they're eating or cooking. Both of these can cause problems. Many people have fallen into these traps and they spend weeks following their calorie goals but not making any progress.

Luckily, in this age of technology, there are many free apps and websites that can help you keep track of all this. There are online recipe nutrition calculators that give you detailed nutrition facts based on the input ingredients and indicated number of servings.

Verywellfit.com has a good recipe nutrition calculator. It couldn't be easier. You can simply copy and paste a list of ingredients into the recipe field and then select the number of servings and it gives you a custom and complete nutrition label.

NOTE: services like these are not fool proof and can commonly have errors. Double check the values they're giving for your ingredients because sometimes they can be way off.

Apps like: MyFitness Pal can be very helpful for quickly checking the caloric value of food and for logging what you've eaten during the day. They offer free food journals where can simply plug in item by item what you're eating throughout the day and it will keep track of everything and show you a running total of calories eaten so far. It will also help you keep track of your calorie targets for each day, and you can even set reminders on your phone so you won't forget to log the food you've eaten.

Exercise:

But what about exercise and activity? It is difficult to pinpoint how many calories you burn through exercise. Again, a lot of this depends on you physiologically and can vary from person to person. There is more reliable data when it comes to cardio exercise. It's more difficult to say how many calories you're burning from weight lifting—partially because different amounts of effort and exertion are required for different people to lift the same amount of weight.

For example: jogging. A fair assumption would be that you're burning about 100-115 calories per mile that you run. Of course, this depends on a lot of factors: how fast are you running, are you running uphill, downhill or on a flat plane etc. These are all just guidelines. If you're running on a treadmill, most of them will track the estimated number of calories you're burning. While they're not completely accurate, it's a good base to go off of.

When it comes to exercise, many people say that unless you're really doing a lot of exercise, you shouldn't deduct it from your calorie intake for the day. This is because of how difficult it can be to calculate the number of calories you're burning and so it's better to just stick the original number of calories and just enjoy the accelerated weight loss you'll experience by augmenting your calorie deficit with exercise.

NOTE: it can certainly be dangerous to exercise when you've consumed too few calories. Indeed, any time you consume too few calories, you could be putting your body at risk. Make sure to consult your physician before starting this diet.

So what can you eat on the Low Calorie Diet?

Here's the good part. You CAN eat anything you want. This is a pretty non-restrictive diet. You're not prohibited from eating carbs or fruit or meat or anything like that. But here's the catch, since you're only allowed a certain number of calories per day, you'll want to choose wisely what you eat.

If you choose to opt for sugary processed calorie dense foods, you'll exceed your daily quota quickly. For example if you go to IHOP and order a stack of sugary pancakes and a fattening omelet filled with cheese and fatty meats and fried in oil and butter, and a sugary Frappuccino, you'll probably almost be at your limit just from one meal.

Whereas if you eat oatmeal and some fresh fruit and eggs, you'll feel just as full, but have consumed a fraction of the calories leaving room for the rest of the meals you'll be eating that day.

What You Can Eat:

As much as you want:
-Fruits and vegetables

In Moderation:

-grains, simple carbs, lean meats, legumes, dairy, fish etc

Rarely:

-calorie dense foods

-heavily processed foods (especially pre-packaged foods and "instant" foods)

-sugars and sugary foods and drinks

-Fatty meats (especially fatty red meats)

-fried foods

-Alcohol

The 2 biggest downfalls here are sugar and fried foods. Sugary foods and fried foods are too calorie dense to even be worth it on a low cal diet. If you get some deep fried chicken tenders, fries and a coke, you'll be basically done for the day because of how highly caloric those foods are. You can eat pretty much anything else in moderation, but you'll really want to severely limit your sugar intake and pretty much eliminate fried food from your diet.

Tips for Success:

It's also important to be on a regular eating schedule and start eating at least some of the same foods regularly. When your eating patterns are sporadic, you'll find it much harder to actually keep track of what you eat, and you may fall far behind in logging your calories. If you eat the same foods regularly, you'll start to remember the caloric value of these foods and it will make your life so much easier. It will help you plan a meal or even a menu for a whole week and you won't need to constantly be typing everything into a nutritional calculator or flipping through calorie book.

Another thing to remember also, is that just like you won't lose all your weight in a day, you won't gain it all back in a day either. Pace yourself, be patient, and don't beat yourself up too much. If you have a bad day or you find out later you miscalculated your calories—or simply it's a special day and you're at an event or attending some type of special occasion, don't worry. You won't "wreck" your progress. Of course, you'll want to keep any "cheat days" few and far between, but don't lose your head if you have an off day, just get back on track the next morning and keep heading towards your goals. You'll get there.

Plus remember, this isn't forever: you're eating a diminished number of calories on purpose to lose weight, but you won't be losing weight forever. Eventually, you'll reach your target weight and be able to increase your caloric intake so that you're merely maintaining instead of losing weight. Always keep that in mind when you're feeling overwhelmed.

Of course, you can still satisfy your sweet tooth—we recommend opting for very small portions of desserts so you still get to satisfy your sweet tooth, but you don't compromise too many calories. But you have to determine if it's worth the sacrifices of calories.

For example: if you're trying to lose a pound a week and you're trying to stay under 1500 calories per day, you may sacrifice 300 calories for ½ cup of ice cream, and it might taste delicious, but it won't be very filling and you'll have only 1200 calories remaining for the entire rest of the day. For some it will be worth it, for others not so much.

A good tip to help you achieve success with this diet is to not try to lose all your weight overnight. Not only is it impossible, but it can be very unhealthy. Try to take it slow and steady. 2-4 pounds of weight loss per month is a very reasonable and means only cutting out 250-500 calories per day. Of course, if you're very overweight, you may be able to lose a lot more weight much more quickly, but again you'll want to consult your doctor first.

One practical piece of advice for how to tackle this diet is by filling up on the healthy low cal stuff and just having a small bit of the unhealthy stuff so you're not miserable. For example, when it's pizza night, instead of cramming six slices into your mouth, have a GIANT bowl of salad and just once slice of pizza. You'll still get to enjoy the pizza, and the salad is very low in calories so you can just keep eating that until you feel full. Then you didn't blow 1500 calories on pizza in one meal.

Another trick is making smart substitutions:

- Grill your meat instead of frying it
- Substitute steamed veggies for rice or pasta
- Use fresh fruit instead of sugar on your cereal or yogurt etc.
- Use skim milk instead of half and half in your coffee
- Sub egg whites for eggs
- Use 0 cal cooking spray instead of oil for sautéing and cooking on the stove top
- Use natural sugar substitutes like Stevia wherever possible

- Drink light beer instead of Craft beer
- Drink clear liquor mixed with soda water with fresh citrus for taste instead of sugary cocktails.
- Lemon and oil salad dressing instead of ranch
- Go bun less on your sandwiches or burgers
- Unsweetened iced tea with lemon instead of sugary sodas
- Fresh fruit with yogurt instead of desserts

Benefits of this diet:

- It's simple, straightforward and very measurable. You pretty much know exactly what you have to do
- Easy to make goals and hold yourself accountable
- Helps you become aware of the nutritional values of food.

Risks:

- Can be too difficult for some people if they're used to eating very highly caloric diets.
- Can make people too obsessed about food
- It can be unhealthy to consume too few calories. Anyone considering this diet should first consult their physician to get clear guidelines

Consensus: if you're someone that gets overwhelmed by all the rules and restrictions of complicated diets and if you have a decent amount of will power, this may be the best choice for you.

If you like to see results and be able to measure and track your success and if you're a big fan of fruits and veggies, you might have great success with this diet.

6. Weight Watchers:

Lose up to 2 pounds a week while still eating ice cream, bacon, cheeseburgers and French fries. Does that sound impossible? Well that's what Weight Watchers claims and many find it to be an effective weight loss solution.

Weight Watchers is one of the most popular, most heavily researched and widely supported diet programs in the world. They have chapters for in-person meetings all across the countries, they offer personal coaching services, they have a massive online community, a robust web presence with success stories, recipes, free info and tips and tons more, and they even have their own magazine. Plus they have cobranded food items you can find all throughout major grocery stores. You can also purchase their meal plans to make your life even easier. Their smart points system is a way to track the food you're eating and represents a lifestyle shift that can help you not only lose weight, but keep the weight off for good.

Smart Points:

Smart points are a proprietary diet tracking tool that Weight Watchers' use to manage their food intake. Weight Watchers is all about the points and not so much about the calorie counting. This makes a lot of sense because not all calories should be treated the same since some calories are just empty with basically no nutritional merit, whereas other calories are full of nutrients that will not only help you feel full, but will improve your health and wellbeing. For example, 200 calories worth of chicken breast and kale salad has much higher nutritional value than 200 calories worth of ice cream (even though it's the same number of calories). And even looking at the differences in portions, you can see how much more sustaining 200 calories of kale and chicken salad will look than 200 calories worth of ice cream. Basically, you're comparing half a scoop of ice cream that probably won't put a dent in your hunger, to a salad that is packed with protein, antioxidants and nutrients that will help fuel you and fill you up. Smart Points takes all this into consideration and assigns food points values based on not only the calorie content, but the nutritional value of the food. The lower the points value, generally the lower in calories and higher in nutrients, whereas the higher in points, generally the higher in calories and lower in nutritional merit.

To better understand how this works, we can use an example: A 300 calorie food would be set at a baseline number of points. Let's pretend it would be set at 10 points. As we discover the nutritional value of this food, we'll be able to adjust our points levels up or down. This food is high in protein, so that means we reduce the number of points for this food. Suddenly, it's only worth 6 points. Vice versa, if it didn't have much protein and was instead high in saturated fat and sugar, we would increase the number of points. Suddenly it's worth 14 points instead of 10.

That was just to illustrate the process, but as you can see, this nuanced way of looking at food takes in the bigger picture. Unlike other diets that simply zero in on one aspect of the food (carbs, calories, fat etc.), this diet takes it all into account and does all the calculating and figuring for you. You don't need to even get into all the nutritional significance, you just need to know how many points a certain food is and then decide accordingly if it's something worth eating.

You're given a daily budget of points based on your body weight. This budget is the total number of points your allowed to consume on a daily basis, and it's all factored and calculated to help you achieve weight loss. For example, if you weight between 200 and 225 lbs, your allotment of points will be somewhere between 24-29 points per day.

Zero Points Foods: yes, you heard right! There are certain foods that are ZERO POINTS! That means that you can basically eat these foods and not do any tracking and you won't use any of your precious allotment of points each day as you consume these foods. Foods like eggs, chicken breast, beans, fish, certain vegetables. Weight Watchers claims to have a list of 200+ Zero Points foods. This should make you breathe a sigh of relief because it means that even if you use up all your Smart Points for the day and are still hungry, you'll still be able to eat more without compromising your diet.

Fit Points: Previously called Active Points which factor into the smart points. Fit Points are points you earn through exercise and physical activity. There are many different ways you could accrue fit points, and also many different ways to track fit points. One of the common ways is by tracking steps through devices like the Fitbit. So, what do you do with your Fit Points? You can eat them. That's right. You can trade in your Fit Points for Smart Points which then increases your daily budget of Smart Points. Fit Points work the opposite of Smart Points in the sense that the more exercise you do, the more Fit Points you get. The alternative to eating your Fit Points is to just eat as normal and enjoy accelerated weight loss. You'll basically be continually eating "under budget" since you're not cashing in your Fit Points, and thus you will lose weight faster because you're burning more calories in your day and not offsetting that deficit by eating more.

Benefits:

Support: it's an incredibly well-thought out, well-supported diet plan. From online communities, to in-person support groups, to personalized coaching, you can have as much support as you choose. There are TONS of resources to help you achieve success in this diet: cookbooks, blogs, prepared food plans, Weight Watchers branded foods in the grocery stores, mobile apps, YouTube video, success stories, testimonials etc. You would be heard pressed to find a Diet program with more support than Weight Watchers.

Real Weight Loss: the whole plan is designed to help you lose weight and really change your entire lifestyle so that you're not only losing weight, but the weight is staying off. They have countless success stories and testimonials of people just like you and me who have achieved great success with the program. These testimonials are a great source of inspiration and help you motivate yourself to achieve the same success.

Flexibility: this program can be as flexible as you want it to be. You can be as involved with coaching and support groups as you want to be, or else you can simply purchase the basic package and do it all on your own. You can be flexible with what you eat, and you can even roll over points if you don't use them all in a day.

No restricted Food Groups: the beauty of this plan is that you can eat ANYTHING you want. Although some foods may have higher points values than others, you can eat anything as long as you can stay within your daily budget. And it's easier than ever because of the Zero Points foods that allow you to eat even after you've exhausted your Smart Points budget. Thus, you can decide as you go how you want to expend your points.

Improved Cardiovascular Health: some clinical trials for Weight Watchers indicated that following the program could contribute to a reduced risk for heart disease. Overcoming obesity and maintaining a healthy body weight is the number one way to prevent heart disease.

Reduced risk of Type 2 Diabetes: By losing weight and maintaining healthy blood sugar levels can reduce your risk of developing insulin resistance which can lead to Type 2 Diabetes.

Risks:

While there aren't many significant risks in following this program, you should always consult your physician first to see if a particular diet regimen is suitable for you.

Cost: some people may find Weight Watchers to be too expensive. Indeed, most other diets on this list are free, so the cost of Weight Watchers may turn some people off. There are different levels of involvement and prices ranging from $150+ per month, to $20 per month. This is dependent on the level of support you require. While some people may see the cost as a worthwhile investment in their health, others will find the cost too much of a burden and will seek alternatives.

Stagnated Weight Loss: some people have experienced stagnated or slow/minimal weight loss. This can especially be the case if you're already at a healthy weight and are just trying to shed those last few pounds to achieve your body goals. The Smart Points and Zero Points ideas are not fool-proof so some experimentation may be required (especially for those last few stubborn pounds), but depending on your goals in dieting, the weight loss may not be rapid enough for you.

As we've Already Stated, there really aren't restrictions on WHAT you can and cannot eat, you'll just want to stay within your daily points budget.

Tips for Success with Weight Watchers:

Drink Water: of course, everyone knows this, but not many people know how important it is. Maintaining good hydration is so important for so many health-related reasons, but especially when it comes to weight loss, drinking a lot of water will help suppress your appetite and will help keep your energy levels up. If you drink a lot of water before a meal, you'll find that you're less "ravenously hungry" as you eat and so you'll eat less. Also, since you're dieting, you'll probably be eating less than you're accustomed to. You may notice a decrease in energy levels (and especially if you're trying to hit the gym a lot, that energy is so important), drinking a lot of water can really help. Often when someone is complaining of fatigue or not enough energy while dieting, the number one reason is because they're dehydrated.

Take full advantage of the support available to you: Weight Watchers has an incredible amount of support options for you. If you're a social person and benefit from a group environment, you'll want to consider joining one of the local chapters and going to meeting. There are also many online communities and you can even get your own personal coach to help you set goals for yourself. There's no end to the possibilities, but accountability is one of the most important parts of solidifying any new habit. Having someone to help keep you accountable will make such a big difference for you. It could mean the difference of binging one night vs making the right choice and working towards your goals. It might be a good motivator for you. If you know that tomorrow you have to meet with your accountability partner, you'll think twice about loading up a bowl of ice cream and plopping down in front of the TV. Also, if you're having strong cravings or are finding it to break out of old habits, having someone to call or talk to can make a huge difference.

Accountability can work great if it goes both ways: this means that you're holding your partner accountable and they're holding you accountable. However, this can only work if you're both really committed to your goals. If you and your partner make each other weaker by allowing each other to indulge too much, then you're probably not the best fit for each other. Sometimes it's better to have a partner that has already made a lot of progress towards their weight loss goals. This will help motivate you, and they can also help show you the ropes and show you what worked for them and what didn't.

Use Your Weekly Points: Weight Watcher's smart point system gives you a daily allotment of points for the food you're consuming, but it also gives you an extra weekly allotment that you can distribute or use as needed throughout the week. This can really help make the diet more bearable for you. This means that you can splurge here and their without wrecking your progress or having to start over. Like any good diet, you'll want to learn moderation. That's what the weekly points are about. That means that you CAN splurge on that cake and ice cream at your coworker's birthday party on Thursday. Of course, you cant do things like that every day, but that's why we call it splurging. It's a rare occurrence reserved for special occasions. As funny as it sounds, having splurges and cheat moments are important to making a diet sustainable. It's very difficult to white knuckle a diet and never give yourself a break and never have a cheat meal. You may be able to do that for a time, but you'll eventually find your resolve slipping and then at some point, you'll throw everything out the window and either binge or just give your diet up all together because you've found it to be too difficult. Sprinkling in a health amount of splurge moments helps reward you for your success and helps remind you that this is lifestyle change—not just a temporary solution. Slow and steady wins the race.

Get Creative With Your Food: the more fun you have with your food and the more you enjoy it, the more you'll become accustomed to your new lifestyle and the less you'll be tempted to fall back on old habits. If you've never been much of a vegetable person, now's your chance to turn over a new leaf. There are so many creative and delicious ways to prepare vegetables—there's no way you could ever get bored. Simply grilling or oven roasting your vegetables with a little olive oil, salt pepper and perhaps some Italian Seasoning can do wonders. You can take sweet potatoes and roast them in the oven, and there you have sweet potato fries that will satisfy your craving for French fries any day. Learn to use herbs and spices and you'll be able to doctor any food up and make anything taste delicious and flavorful.

Get Rid of Temptations: Although it may go against your better nature to throw food out, do it. Just see the money you've "lost" as an investment in your health. The boxes of oreos, the cartons of ice cream, the bags of frozen chicken nuggets etc. You will have enough temptation outside your home, the least you can do is to turn your home into a relatively temptation-free zone. It's a funny thing about getting rid of junk food: if you don't have it, you won't eat it. In a lot of ways, it's that simple. If you don't have it easily accessible (in your freezer, in your cupboards, in your pantry), you won't eat it. In many ways, it's out of sight and out of mind. Of course you can't as easily control the environment outside of your house, and luckily you have those weekly points to expend on temptations and cravings that are just too good to pass up. However, we advise that you reserve those splurge moments for outside of the home. Get rid of the junk in your house and stop buying it when you go to the grocery store. You'll be AMAZED at the results. If you're afraid you won't be able to resist filling your cart with junk when you go to the store, I have 3 practical tips for you that will help you stay on track.

- Take a list: I mean it. Make a thorough shopping list (only putting things you're really allowed to eat), and stick to that list. Go into the store and don't even look at the shelves. Just go in, grab what's on your list and get out.
- Don't Shop alone: get your accountability partner to go with you, or take along a family member or friend who will help keep you accountable.
- Don't Shop Hungry: we make irrational decisions when we're hungry, so make sure you never go grocery shopping when you're hungry. If you normally shop after work, postpone your shopping trip until after dinner. You'll find you're better able to make level headed decisions when your stomach isn't screaming for attention.

Get Your Steps In: get moving one way or the other. Most of us unfortunately do not have jobs that allow us to be super active throughout the day. What this means is that many of us spend the day sitting all day, and we have to actively seek out ways to build activity into our day. It could be something as simple as going for a walk on your lunch break, or as intense as committing to a one hour workout 4 days a week either before or after work. Although working out isn't necessary for weight loss, it's extremely important for your mental and physical health and when used to supplement a good diet, it can super charge your weight loss.

The most important thing to remember here is to find something that you actually enjoy doing. If you hate jogging then maybe don't force yourself to jog every day. Maybe swimming is more your thing, or maybe you're more the type of person who prefers to get exercise through sports. Take up tennis, or join an adult volleyball league. Maybe you're a nature lover. Combine exercise with the great outdoors by going hiking. Maybe you're a Netflix addict. Step on the treadmill and crank up the incline and

and speed and do some brisk walking while catching up on a favorite show on your iPad. The possibilities are endless. Just pick something you like or can at least tolerate doing, and you'll find it much easier to implement and sustain an exercise habit in your daily life.

There are many, many other strategies and helpful tips for success with Weight Watchers. The Weight Watchers online community is overflowing with helpful tips and tricks—especially when it comes to forming better cooking and eating habits.

Consensus: if you're the type of person that benefits from support and community and the idea of having points assigned to you is appealing, Weight Watchers might be your golden ticket. If you don't mind the cost and are not concerned with understanding the tracking all the nutritional significance of the diet and making it your own, then the Weight Watchers program is a program that makes it very easy for you.

In a Nutshell: Consistently hailed as one of the healthiest diets in the world, the DASH Diet is a holistic and balanced diet that is high in fruits, vegetables, whole grains, and lean proteins, and low in fat. The DASH diet works particularly well with controlling hypertension and reducing sodium intake.

What is the DASH Diet?

The word DASH comes from the acronym Dietary Approaches to Stop Hypertension. In the year 1992, the National Heart, Lung and Blood Institute (NHLBI) conducted a research study seeking ways to reduce critical blood pressure and cardiovascular health problems in the United States. The DASH study involved doctors, nutritionists and other medical representatives from the top 5 health Centre's of US.

The original research resulted in forming a wholesome nutrition plan known as Dash Diet that helped people in reducing their high blood pressure (or hypertension).

Researchers from various institutes concluded that the Dash diet was one of the best plans to adopt if you have one of the four problems,

1.) Blood Pressure

2.) Cholesterol

3.) Diabetes

4.) Weight issues

How does the DASH Diet work?

The food plan focuses on fruits, vegetables, non-fat/low-fat dairy and whole grains such as cereals. The eating plan also includes the consumption of high fiber foods, medium to low amounts of fat, low red meat, and less sugar. An additional benefit of this diet is that it is rich in different vitamins and minerals that are important in achieving a healthy body.

Another good thing about this diet plan is that it lowers your sodium intake in your diet (daily consumption for sodium is only 2,3oo mg on the dash diet) that will help regulate blood pressure levels. That's because studies show that eating food with high sodium content could lead to a spike in blood pressure.

The diet plan has claimed to lower the blood pressure in just two weeks and has been recommended by Centers for Disease Control, American Heart Association, The National Heart, Lung, and Blood Institute, the Mayo Clinic, US Government guidelines for treatment of high blood pressure and a lot more.

Benefits of the DASH Diet

Aside from lowering blood pressure and helping you lose weight, several studies also claim that it can prevent other diseases such as cancer, stroke, heart failure, diabetes, kidney stones, and osteoporosis.

For diabetes, the high-fiber food consumption that is part of the DASH Diet (minimum intake is about 30g of fiber daily) does not only help promote better digestive health, but it can also control glucose and insulin production; which also makes it a great food plan for diabetics.

The other advantages of the DASH diet are: reversing ageing effects, strengthening the bones, joints and muscles, rejuvenating the hair and skin, reducing cholesterol levels, cutting the risk factor of metabolic syndrome, and improving heart health. Exercise or regular workouts are recommended with the DASH Diet in order to reap further health benefits.

Remember, this diet is not just any fad diet. This is not the type of diet where: once you achieved your health/weight goals in "x" amount of time, you will quit the diet. The point of the diet is an overall lifestyle change to be maintained for a healthier you.

Anyone who makes a change to their diet will experience the symptoms of that change. The experience will be different for everyone because people come to the DASH diet from unique starting points in terms of diet quality and composition. However, knowing that your mind and body need to adjust to change will help you keep moving forward.

Best Foods to Eat on the DASH Diet

The following are the best foods you can eat while on the DASH diet. These are foods that are high in fiber, magnesium, potassium, and other vitamins and minerals. This is not meant to be a comprehensive list, rather this is meant to give you some good ideas for what you should be eating while on the DASH diet.

Vegetables

While following the DASH diet, you should be consuming around 4-5 servings of vegetables per day. We all know that vegetables are good for us and that they are very healthy foods, yet I think few of us realize just how healthy vegetables really are:

Eating vegetables regularly can help to reduce the risk of heart disease and stroke (5).

It can help protect you against certain types of cancer (6).

- Vegetables are low in calories and high in fiber. This means that you can eat as many of them as you want and not have to worry about overeating. And the fiber will help to keep you fuller for a longer period of time as well as ensure proper bowel movements. (this generally applies to non-starchy vegetables. Vegetables like corn and potatoes should generally be eaten in moderation since they are higher in calories and carbohydrates.)

- Vegetables are very nutrient dense, meaning that they contain a lot of nutrients even though they're low in overall calories. Something like a candy bar, on the other hand, isn't nutrient dense. It contains a lot of calories, but it has very few nutrients.

- Folic acid: folic acid helps the body to create red blood cells. Red blood cells are necessary for transporting oxygen throughout your body. Getting proper amounts of folic acid is especially important for pregnant women or women who plan on becoming pregnant to ensure proper fetal development.

- Vegetables are rich in so many vitamins and minerals! Vegetables contain high amounts of vitamin A, C, potassium, iron, magnesium, and calcium.

- Vegetables are delicious. Very few foods are as versatile in how you can prepare them. If you think vegetables taste boring, you're doing it wrong.

There are so many ways you can dress your vegetables up and make them taste shockingly delicious.

Here's a list of vegetables that you should consume on the DASH diet:

- Sweet potatoes
- Tomatoes
- Squash
- Spinach
- Potatoes
- Lima Beans
- Kale
- Green Beans
- Peas
- Collard Greens
- Mustard Greens
- Broccoli
- Cauliflower
- Carrots

Fruits

Just like vegetables, fruits are very good for you and will provide you with many of the same vitamins and minerals that vegetables will. Unfortunately, fruits sometimes get a bad reputation because they contain fructose, which is a type of sugar. The thing is though that fructose is a natural sugar, not a processed sugar, and the benefits you'll receive from eating fruits far outweighs the fact that they contain some sugar in them.

While following the DASH diet eating plan, you'll want to consume 4-5 servings of fruit per day. Here are some of the amazing benefits of eating fruit:

- Fruits contain low amounts of sodium, calories, and fat.

- Similar to vegetables, fruit is very nutrient dense. So basically, you'll be getting a good bang-for-your-buck when it comes to getting the most nutrients for the least amount of calories. Eating rich nutrient dense foods is critical for your success with the DASH diet.

- Fruits can help to lower cholesterol levels as well as reduce the risk for heart disease (7).

- Additionally, fruits contain high amounts of vitamin A and C, potassium, magnesium, folic acid, and fiber.

- Fruits also contain high amounts of water, which will help to keep your body hydrated.

- Some fruits and especially berries are seen as "superfoods" for their antioxidant properties. Consumption of these fruits have been linked to reduction in risks for certain cancers and other types of diseases.

Here's a list of fruits you should consume on the DASH diet:

- Raisins
- Blueberries
- Raspberries
- Strawberries
- Peaches
- Pineapples
- Melons
- Grapes
- Apples
- Apricots
- Bananas
- Dates
- Oranges
- Grapefruit
- Mangoes
- Tangerines

Dairy

While on the DASH diet eating plan, you should be consuming around 2-3 servings of dairy per day. It's important to note that you'll want to be eating low-fat dairy. The DASH diet limits certain types of fat intake, and consuming large amounts of fat through dairy isn't ideal, especially if it can be avoided in the first place. Here are some of the key benefits of consuming dairy in your diet:

- Dairy is high in protein. Protein is one of three macronutrients (carbs and fat being the other two), and it's responsible for aiding in many of your body's functions. One of the main things protein does is rebuild and repair tissue.

- It's an important building block for muscle, bone, skin, cartilage, and blood. It's also needed for the growth of hair and nails. So needless to say, protein is a very critical nutrient regardless if you're looking to pack on muscle or not.

- Dairy is rich in calcium. When you think of strong bones, what do you think of? You probably think of some kid or adult drinking a glass of milk. We've really been bombarded with the fact that milk (and other dairy products for that matter) is good for strong bones, and it really is so true! This is all because of calcium. Calcium is necessary for maintaining bone mass in the body, which helps to support the skeleton.

- Skim Milk

- 1% Milk

- Low-Fat Cheese

- Low-Fat Cottage Cheese

- Low-Fat Yogurt

This is one of the many differentiators of the DASH diet vs. other diets. One of the biggest issues with so many other diets out there is that there's a calcium deficiency. Medical professionals are always criticizing the leading diets for this. In the short-term it may not cause many problems, but long term it can lead to pre-mature aging, bone deterioration and other diseases. With the DASH diet, you won't have to worry about that. You'll probably even be consuming more calcium than you previously were. This is one of the things I really love about the DASH diet. It's so balanced. It's not trying to just focus on one thing—it helps you improve your health holistically with minimal side effects.

Meats, Poultry, and Fish

You'll also be consuming some meat on the DASH diet plan. Meat isn't as heavily emphasized as some of the other food groups, such as fruits and vegetables however, it's still an important part of the diet regime. You'll want to consume around 1-2 servings of meat, poultry, and/or fish per day.

- Poultry
- Fish
- Bison
- Venison
- Beef

Nuts, Seeds, and Dried Beans

You'll want to consume 3 servings of various nuts, seeds, and dried beans per week on the DASH diet. You'll be eating quite a bit less of this food group compared to some of the other food groups, and it's for a good reason. Nuts are comprised mostly of fat.

Yes, there are good types of fat and bad types of fat (more on this later), however fat contains 9 calories per gram. On the other hand, protein and carbs only contain 4 calories per gram of food. This means that you'll be consuming over twice the amount of calories for the same amount of food if you're consuming fat. Those calories can add up rather quickly, and this is something we want to be aware of.

That's why you'll only be consuming 3 servings per week of these different nuts, seeds, and dried beans. As I just mentioned though, there is such a thing as good fat and bad fat. Bad fats would be something like trans-fat and saturated fat. Excessive amounts of these types of fat have been shown to increase the risk for heart disease as well as other health problems (12).

Nuts and seeds, on the other hand, contain mono and polyunsaturated fats. These are a healthy type of fat that can help to lower your risk of heart disease by decreasing your low-density lipoproteins (LDL) and maintaining your high-density lipoproteins (HDL). Your LDL's are the bad type of cholesterol, and your HDL's are the good kind of cholesterol.

The reality is that consuming too many calories overall from all three macronutrients (protein, carbs, and fat) is bad for us and that's what leads to weight gain. Yes, certain types of fat should be limited or avoided altogether (such as saturated or trans-fat), but that's not to say that all fat is bad for you because that simply isn't the case. Here are some of the benefits of consuming nuts, seeds, and dried beans:

- They are a rich source of energy. As I talked about earlier, fat contains 9 calories per gram. This can be dangerous if overeaten, however you have to remember why we're eating food in the first place—to get energy! Our body needs daily energy to maintain itself and carry out its daily functions.
- Contain healthy amounts of magnesium and fiber. Are you starting to notice a common theme here? Many of the foods you'll be consuming on the DASH diet are rich in magnesium! It's such a key mineral for getting and staying healthy, especially if you have hypertension.

- Almonds
- Hazelnuts
- Mixed Nuts
- Peanuts
- Walnuts
- Sunflower Seeds
- Natural Peanut Butter
- Natural Almond Butter
- Kidney Beans
- Lentils
- Split Peas

Fats and Oils

Fats and oils are another essential part of the DASH diet. Again, fats have gotten a bad reputation over the years, but it isn't all justified. The same goes for oils. When you think of oily food, what do you typically think of? Probably something that's greasy, fried, contains a lot of fat, and is unhealthy for you right?

Whole Grains

On the DASH eating plan, you're going to want to consume 6-8 servings of whole grains per day. It's very important to note that you'll want to be consuming whole grains here and not refined grains. Refined grains are more processed than whole grains and thus lose vitamins, minerals, and fiber during the process which means you'll basically just be consuming empty calories when consuming refined grains.

Whole grains, on the other hand, contain more vitamins and fiber, which is key to keeping you fuller longer. Whole grains still contain all three parts of the grain, which are the bran, germ, and endosperm.

When refined grains get processed, they're stripped of the bran and germ, which contain many key nutrients. Not only that, but whole grains are rich in things such as thiamin, riboflavin, niacin, and folate. These are part of the B vitamins complex.

Here's a list of acceptable whole grains should you eat while on the DASH diet:

- Whole-wheat pasta
- Whole-wheat bread
- Brown rice
- Whole-grain cereal
- Oats

Foods You'll Want to Limit on the DASH Diet

Processed foods:

Processed foods are made with certain ingredients that will extend the shelf life of those foods. On one hand, this seems great. It allows the expiration date of a food item to be extended longer so we can take a longer time to eat the food if we wish.

However, we have to take a step back and consider the harmful effects these ingredients can have on our bodies over the long haul. Here are some reasons why you'll want to limit the consumption of processed foods:

Empty Calories

Processed foods in most cases contain a lot of empty calories. Imagine eating broccoli for example. This vegetable is rich in a lot of key vitamins and nutrients that your body needs. It doesn't contain a lot of calories, and the calories that it does contain are jam-packed with healthy nutrients.

On the flip side, consider a processed food item such as a candy bar. The candy bar doesn't contain very many beneficial vitamins and minerals for our bodies. It also contains a lot of calories from simple sugars. That's why the calories from something like a candy bar are considered to be empty. They're providing your body with nothing useful that it needs.

So, you'll likely be unable to get full and stay satisfied, meaning that you'll have to eat even more calories. This is why you must be cautious when eating processed foods. The calories won't do much to keep you full, and it can be very easy to overeat them.

Trans-fats and Processed Oils

Remember that on the DASH diet we are seeking to eliminate or greatly limit the amount of trans fat that we're consuming. Most processed foods contain quite a bit of trans fat and processed oils that we'll want to avoid. These kinds of fats are high in Omega-6 fatty acids.

Omega-6 fatty acids by themselves are not bad, however they can become a problem when consumed in excess compared to Omega-3 fatty acids. Omega-6 fatty acids cause our bodies to become inflamed. Excess inflammation can cause damage to our joints, impede recovery, and cause heart disease among other things (14).

This is why it's important to have a balance of Omega-3 fatty acids, which act as an anti-inflammatory in the body. The Omega-3 fatty acids can help to counteract the inflammation from the Omega-6 fatty acids.

Foods too Low in Fiber

Processed foods contain a low amount of fiber. Other foods like fruits and vegetables contain high amounts of fiber. As I mentioned earlier, fiber is not only important for our digestive health, but it's also very important for keeping us full for longer periods of time.

This is the real danger of eating too many processed foods. They don't fill you up very well, so you have to eat more of them to get full. This likely means that you'll eat more calories than you should have.

Too many simple carbohydrates: Some people think that you should avoid carbs at all costs, and it's easy to believe considering how bad of a reputation carbs have been getting lately. However, all of this hate on carbs isn't justified. There are good carbs and bad carbs.

Not all carbs are evil and should be avoided like the plague. There are two different kinds of carbohydrates—simple and complex. Simple carbs are carbs that are quickly broken down and processed by the body. This is a bad thing because the rapid breakdown leads to a spike in your insulin levels.

Insulin spikes can lead to food cravings at random times, and your body doesn't burn fat while your insulin levels are high (15).

Conversely, there are complex carbohydrates. These are carbs such as brown rice and sweet potatoes. These kinds of carbs are slower digesting carbs that will not cause spikes in your blood sugar levels. Complex carbs are considered to be healthy carbs (in moderation of course). They also contain many beneficial vitamins and nutrients.

Juices Sodas and Other Artificially Sweetened Beverages

Wait what? I thought things like orange juice were good for you? Yes, if you took oranges, squeezed them, and only drank the juice that came directly from the oranges that would be ok in moderation (although that'd be the equivalent of eating several oranges, so you'd want to factor that in to your daily servings of fruit).

However, most fruit juices and other artificially sweetened beverages aren't healthy options. The main reason is because they are loaded with a bunch of excessive sugar. Most juices don't contain purely the sugar found in the fruits.

Most of the time, there's added sugar in the juices. Yes, these juices do contain a lot of vitamins such as vitamin A and C, however this doesn't make them a healthy drink option. In fact, this deceives people into thinking that it's a healthy choice when the truth is that it's not.

If you want to get more vitamin A and C in your diet, then eat more fruits and vegetables. You don't have to go out of your way by drinking more fruit juices to get more vitamins. Yes, it's easier to consume these vitamins by drinking them, but it comes at a cost. And that cost is excessive amounts of sugar.

White Bread and White Carbs

On the DASH diet, you're going to consuming whole grains, such as whole-wheat bread. Something you'll want to avoid is white bread. On the surface, it might appear as if bread is bread so what's the big deal with white bread? Why do we want to avoid eating it whenever possible?

For starters, white bread is a simple carbohydrate. As I mentioned earlier, simple carbs should be avoided in favor of complex carbs. Simple carbohydrates provide little nutritional value to your body, and they also cause rapid spikes in your blood sugar levels, which can lead to food cravings at random times throughout the day.

Not only that, but white bread ranks high on the glycemic index scale (GI scale for short). The GI scale measures how fast or slow different carbohydrates cause increases in blood glucose levels. The slower the carbohydrate increases blood glucose levels, the better it is, and thus the lower the score it'll receive on the glycemic index scale.

The scale ranges from 0-100, and basically what you need to know is that the closer a food item is to 0, the better it is for you. White bread has a GI score of 75 (18), which isn't good at all. It'll quickly raise blood sugar levels much faster than other carbohydrates will. That's why on the DASH diet, you'll be consuming whole grains, which rank much lower on the glycemic index scale. And you'll want to greatly limit or completely avoid carbs such as white bread. This includes white bread, white rice, white pasta etc.

Fried Foods

Frying food drastically increases the amount of fat content in the food. Often fried food is seasoned with an excessive amount of salt. This will unnecessarily increase the amount of sodium in the food. And as you learned earlier, taking in too much sodium can cause hypertension, which is why you'll want to limit sodium intake on the DASH diet.

And since Fried foods contain a lot of added fat, this means that they contain an excessive amount of calories as well.

Cookies, Cakes, and Other Pastries

These sweet treats are another simple carbohydrate that you'll want to watch out for. Their nutritional content is made up primarily of refined sugars and other processed ingredients. These foods usually contain shortening, which is a type of solid fat that's high in saturated fat. This is one of the bad types of fat that you'll want to limit whenever possible. Yes, these foods are tasty, but be wary not to over consume them as part of your 5 servings per week following the nutritional plan

Why the DASH Diet Really Works:

The Dash Diet is known for being a FAMILY-oriented Diet. It can be adopted by individuals of all ages right from kids to adults to the older members, this nutrition plan takes care of the overall health of the family. Of course always consult your doctor before starting any new diet plan and of course if Children are involved you'll want to clear it with their Pediatrician.

1.) A Wholesome Diet

Dash Diet promotes consuming all three macronutrients – carbs, proteins and fats. The idea behind the diet is to take care of your primary meals – breakfast, lunch and dinner along with your snacking needs throughout the day. In a diet like this you tend to eat all kinds of healthy foods which in turn reduces your chance/desire of eating junk or unhealthy food items.

2.) Take Control of Your Blood Pressure

Life these days is stressful and it can get really difficult to stick to a meal plan, let alone a nutrition plan. The consumption of whole grains, fruits and vegetables help in reducing hunger especially when taken in small quantities throughout the day. Potassium, calcium and magnesium filled foods work as crucial elements to stabilize the levels of blood pressure.

Now, many people are unclear about the quantities of sodium that our body requires. So, you may ask me, isn't sodium as important as the other elements of nutrition?

Well, yes, it is! Sodium is an essential element for our body and our sodium intake is a concern more than a question. The Dash Diet is designed in a way that it gives you the right amount of sodium which eases critical body functions and does not allow additional fluids to increase. High amounts of sodium can cause extra fluids to build which in turn raises your blood pressure.

The NIH has revealed that the Dash Diet can bring down an individual's blood pressure in JUST 14 days – Amazing Fact

3.) The NEW Added Benefit of the Dash Diet – Cholesterol Management

For some reason, the Dash Diet is known to be one of the MOST RESEARCHED topics of its kind. Researchers found out that this diet does not just help you lower your BP but also supports you in managing your cholesterol levels. How, you may ask? Fibers play a significant role in managing one's cholesterol levels. The foods consumed as per Dash nutrition plans includes whole wheat items such as brown rice, oats, barley, millet and similar others which are a great source of fiber.

Recently, there was an interesting twist in a Dash study which stated that the consumption of high-fat dairy products in the diet could actually lower bad cholesterol levels in individuals who were affected. Hey! Hang on there, before you call me nuts for contradicting myself let me tell you something: in addition to the new findings it was also noticed that two individuals who followed the Dash diet with two different patterns of consuming high-fat and low-fat dairy products got the same results of reduced blood pressure. Now, that's what I call the magic of DASH!!

Health Tip: The proper fiber portion for men can range from 30 to 38 grams per day whereas for women it could be between 20 to 25 grams per day.

4.) The Weight Management Plan

The Dash Diet has emerged as a weight loss plan over the period of years and is said to have a great impact on individuals who are struggling with weight issues such as obesity. There is no denial that apart from its prime motive of minimizing heart problems by reducing your blood pressure the Dash Diet has measurable effects on one's weight. The consumption of fruits and vegetables at regular intervals keeps you full and in turn helps you keep a check on your calorie intake. However, if you are looking for a quick overnight weight loss solution, you may be out of luck. This is a slow and steady process that will contribute to overall better health as well as significant weight loss.

Dash Diet for Weight Loss

Even though this dieting plan was created for the primary purpose of lowering blood pressure and getting a handle on cholesterol, we're going to adapt it in a way that also makes it a powerful weight-loss tool. This dieting plan already puts an emphasis on eating food that is low in cholesterol and saturated fat. The fact that it will have you eating more whole foods will lead to a certain amount of weight-loss automatically.

What we're going to do is take the DASH diet and make a few minor tweaks to make it more efficient for losing weight.

Keep a Food Journal

Having a food journal gives you an easy way to go back to review your food consumption periodically. Write down every meal you eat and place a timestamp on it. This includes snacks and drinks–everything you put into your body should be documented. Take it a step further and document your activity while eating. For example, "I had popcorn while watching a movie."

It's easy to lose track of your food consumption, so documenting it gives you an easy way to go back and review it on a weekly basis. You can see where you stand in terms of your eating habits, so you can start fixing the bad ones.

Calculate Your Calorie Goal

If you are planning to lose weight, then you will have to lower your calorie intake, so that it's less than what you burn on a daily basis. But you must do it gradually so that it doesn't throw your metabolism out of whack.

Start out by determining exactly what activities you perform on a daily basis.

When you determine how many calories you are burning per day, then you need to develop a plan. Here's an example:

You are burning 1,200 calories per day, so you will set up a list of goals as follows:

Week 1: 2,000 calories per day.

Week 2: 1,600 calories per day.

The primary goal of the diet is not actually for weight loss, but with the demand for an effective diet plan that can also solve different health problems, a new DASH Diet research has been conducted to further optimize the present diet plan. Carbs that are not nutritionally balanced were eliminated and more protein-rich food and heart healthy fats were added in the diet, resulting in an effective weight loss diet plan. There are two phases in the diet. Phase One is for the first 14 days of the diet, while Phase Two comes in after 2 weeks in the diet.

Phase 1: Shed Weight Two Weeks

During these 14 days you will learn how to satisfy your hunger with DASH Diet approved foods and as a result, you will feel fuller for a longer time. While whole grains, starchy veggies and fruits are included in the DASH Diet, it's advised that you eliminate these food groups first in the first two weeks of the diet; doing this will help regulate your blood sugar levels and will also curb your cravings for food. Milk is should also be avoided, but you can however, get at least moderated servings of non-fat yogurt. (Don't worry, you'll be able to re-introduce these foods back into your diet in moderate quantities later).

Amp up your consumption of green veggies such as spinach or other vegetables like broccoli, or cabbage, as well as other vegetables such as cucumbers, peppers and tomatoes.

You can also enjoy up to six ounces of lean meats, fish and poultry a day. Aim for four to five servings of beans or lentils a week.

Be wise in choosing your sources of fat. The best way to do this is by eating fish rich in healthy fats such as salmon and mackerel, or by using oils such as olive oil, and almond oil. Absolutely avoid foods that contain saturated and trans fats such as whole-fat dairy, fried foods, vegetable shortening, and store-bought pastries.

Phase 2: Kick It Up a Notch!

After the first 14 days, you will continue eating the foods from Phase 1 but you may start eating some other healthy foods that will help you continue your weight loss. You any choose the following food groups:

Whole Grains: Choose from breads and pasta, cereals, or any items made with whole grain. And totally eliminate foods made from refined grains such as white bread and pasta because these foods cause your blood sugar levels to spike. You can have six to eight servings of whole grains a day.

Fruit: Either fresh or frozen, you should aim to consume four to five servings of fruits daily.

Low-Fat Milk or Yogurt: These are great sources of calcium and Vitamin D. for your body in order to give you strong muscles and bones and also keep your metabolism working.

Sugar-Sugar and other sweets are now allowed in this phase as long as you limit it to not more than five servings a day.

Alcohol- alcohol in the form of wine is allowed in phase two as long as you limit it to a small glass occasionally.

If you really want to live and healthy for the rest of your life, I suggest the you follow the meal plan in phase two and you'll see that you'll be reaping the benefits of DASH Diet in no time.

Make the Transition Slowly

When you make too many changes all at once, you will destabilize your body. This makes you crave your old diet and leads to relapses. It's extremely difficult to fight off your body's survival instincts, and that's exactly what your body does when it's in shock. It believes that survival is at risk, so it creates irresistible urges.

That's why it's important to make the transition slowly. Pace yourself by adapting to your new dietary plan so that your body doesn't even notice. You will eventually experience a full change and wonder how you ever led an unhealthy lifestyle.

Reduce Your Consumption of Fat and Sugar Even Further

Even though the DASH diet is going to have you reducing trans and saturated fat intake, in order to lose weight, you will need to avoid/reduce all types of fat in the beginning. Once you have reached your weight goal, then you can gradually work your way back up to the normal fats.

Stick to poultry and fish as your primary sources of meat. You should probably limit meat to once every day. Replace it with vegetables that are high in protein.

You will also need to reduce the sugars that you consume, including fruits in the beginning, if you want to lose weight. You should limit fruit consumption to one serving per day. Take a multi-vitamin to make up for the loss of nutrients. Once you have reached your weight loss goal, you can start to enjoy fruits as normal again.

Limit Sodium to 1,500 mg per Day

Remember when I said there were two types of DASH diet plans? You are going to want to opt for the one with less sodium intake. This is an area where so many people mess up when losing weight. They do everything right, except keeping their sodium intake down. Then they don't lose weight because the sodium causes their body to retain more water.

The main way to lower your sodium is by avoiding meats that are high in sodium. You will need to pay close attention to labels.

Eat More Vegetables and Whole Grains

Weight loss requires a few additional steps, one of which is to eat even more vegetables. Since you will need to reduce meat and sugar consumption in the initial stages, you will have to replace them with vegetables and whole grains. When I say whole grains, I mean everything–rice and noodles included.

Again, when using canned vegetables be sure that you read the label because some of those items are loaded with sodium and added sugar. Just keep in mind that you need to make these changes gradually to avoid shocking your system.

Fat-Free is Not Always Healthy

Fat-free does not always mean that a product is healthy. For example, some fat-free salad dressings contain even more calories than their fat-filled counterparts! That's why it's so important to read labels.

Most people will just blindly trust that the words "fat-free" mean healthier. That is simply not always the case.

Distribute Your Calories Throughout the Day

Eating smaller portions of food throughout the entire day will help your body burn calories more efficiently because of the metabolic boost that accompanies it. If you are eating a super large dinner, then spread that meal throughout the entire day. Usually, people who eat huge dinners skip lunch, which is a huge mistake.

Eating smaller portions is the absolute best habit you can develop for losing weight. Just this one change makes a huge difference. You should follow a specific meal pattern. The more consistent you are, the more efficient your body will function.

- Breakfast
- Morning snack
- Lunch
- Afternoon snack
- Dinner
- After-dinner snack (at least two hours before bed)

One of the final weight-loss tips for adding to the DASH diet is to exercise regularly, so the next chapter is dedicated to exercise.

Exercise Plan

Now we're going to move onto a topic that drives so many people away from their weight-loss plans, but let me share a secret that you will not hear from other so-called experts:

You do not have to exercise to lose weight!

Exercise is optional, but it is highly recommended due to its many health benefits. But working out on its own is not enough to live a healthy lifestyle. Healthy eating is always the first and only required step. So, I want you to look at exercise as an added bonus and not a requirement. That mindset will create realistic expectations on your part so that if you happen to miss a day of exercise, then you won't completely give up like so many others.

Weight-loss only requires you to create a calorie deficit, so you can choose any method you want as long as you are accomplishing that goal.

You cannot out-exercise a bad diet!

Consumption plays the biggest role in creating a calorie deficit. There are also other factors involved, including stress, sleep habits, and lifestyle choices. The truth is that the journey to a healthier lifestyle is a personal one that does not look the same for every person. What worked for those Internet "experts" might not work for you, and that's okay. So rather than allowing them to rip up your hopes and dreams, find your own path.

Keeping all of that in mind, exercise comes with a ton of benefits that will help you live a more productive life. So now that we understand that exercise shouldn't be placed on some unrealistic pedestal, let's dive deeper into the subject.

- Food choices are more important than workout choices.
- Exercise should become a meaningful part of your routine.
- If you exercise, you have to push yourself.

- You must find exercises that you enjoy; otherwise, you will skip them.

So, you have the right expectations now, and we have set a lot of Internet opinions straight, so let's look at some actual workouts that you can do. While we're focusing on exercises that burn the most calories in the shortest amount of time, you are free to find other options if they fit your lifestyle better.

Consensus: one of the most balanced and wholesome diets out there, the DASH diet can make a huge difference particularly if you struggle with hypertension. If weight loss is your primary goal, the traditional DASH Diet may not be robust enough for you. Consult your physician to see if this diet is the right approach to help you achieve your goals.

8). The Alkaline Diet:

The Alkaline diet is also called the alkaline ash diet, acid ash diet, alkaline acid diet, or acid alkaline diet. This is actually a group of diets loosely related to each other. The main idea is that there are certain foods that directly affect the pH and acidity of the body's fluids, such as the blood and urine. This effect is believed to be therapeutic for certain health issues.

The Basics

The body has its own regulatory mechanism for balancing pH or its acid-base condition. The alkaline diet claims to help or boost this function. The traditional concept of the alkaline diet is to avoid eating poultry, meats, grains and cheese. The goal is to make the urine less acidic and more alkaline. This means increasing the urine's pH level. This is believed to help prevent the recurrence of UTIs (urinary tract infections) and discourage the formation of kidney stones (nephrolithiasis).

When eating foods, the body burns them to extract calories or energy. The extracted energy will then be used by the cells. If not, then some of these will be stored. This burning process is a slow and well-controlled one. So, when something gets burned, a residue is produced. It's like burning wood and ash is left behind. This ash is classified as either alkaline or acidic.

The Alkaline Diet was developed with the help of the US National Institute of Health as a means to lower blood pressure without the need for medication. Aside from being able to lower blood pressure, the Alkaline Diet has also proven to lower the risk of other diseases such as stroke, heart failure, diabetes, cancer, osteoporosis, and kidney stones. Not only will it work for you today, it's designed in such a way that it will have long term effects—so you can be sure that you'll be able to live a long and healthy life.

The Alkaline Diet is comprised of low-fat or non-fat dairy, fruits, vegetables, lean meats, whole grains, poultry, fish, beans, and nuts that are filled with various vitamins and minerals such as potassium, magnesium and calcium that your body certainly needs to develop and function. It is a diet that is high in fiber and low in fat so it would be easy for you to lose weight and lower your cholesterol levels and it also aims to reduce the amount of sodium that you consume so the systems of the body can be stabilized. This way, you can live your life the best way possible. Aside from eating the right kinds of food, it is also recommended that you lessen or quit smoking and exercise regularly so you can be sure that you'll be able to maintain your ideal weight and that a lot of diseases can be prevented.

If you choose to follow the ALKALINE diet, your systolic blood pressure will be able to drop by at least 7 to 12 points, which is a big help for your cholesterol levels to go down and make sure that you would not be suffering from any heart ailments or strokes anytime soon.

According to the diet, the acidity or alkalinity of the ash will have an effect on the body. Acidic ash will cause the body's fluids to become more acidic. Alkaline ash will cause the body's fluid pH to become more alkaline. Eating foods that produce neutral ash will have no effect on the body.

Acid ash is believed to increase the body's vulnerability to certain diseases. Alkaline ash is considered to have protective effects on the body. By eating more alkaline ash-producing foods, the body becomes "alkalinized" and health improves.

The premise of this diet is that different kinds of foods have different effects in the body. Meats, grains, poultry, eggs, fish and cheese produce acid ash in the body. Vegetables and fruits, with the exception of plums, prunes and cranberries, produce alkaline ash. The designation of alkaline or acid ash depends on the effect of the food residue after combustion happens and not on the actual acidity of the food.

For example, citrus foods are known as acidic but in the alkaline diet, these are considered alkaline-producing foods because the residue has an alkalizing effect in the body.

The components of food determine whether the residue becomes acidic or alkaline. Components such as sulfur, phosphate and protein will leave acidic ash residue. Food components like calcium, potassium and magnesium will leave alkaline ash residue.

Food groups considered as acidic, neutral or alkaline include:

Acidic food group: eggs, dairy, fish, poultry, meats, alcohol and grains

Neutral food group: natural fats, sugars and starches

Alkaline food groups: nuts, vegetables, legumes and fruits

What is the body's pH and how is it regulated?

The body's pH refers to how acidic or alkaline the body fluids are. The pH range is:

Acidic: pH 0 to 6.99

Neutral: pH 7

Alkaline: pH 7.11 to 14

In the body, different fluids have different pH levels. It isn't uniform. For instance, the stomach is naturally acidic, even if there is no food. It becomes more acidic around mealtimes, contributing to the feelings of hunger. The acidity comes from the stomach acids, particularly HCl (hydrochloric acid). The normal stomach pH is 2 to 3.5, a highly acidic condition. Acidity is not always a bad thing in the body. The highly acidic environment of the stomach is necessary for digestion because it aids in breaking down tough food components.

The blood, on the other hand, needs a more alkaline environment. It normally has a pH of 7.35 to 7.45, which is in a slightly alkaline range. The blood pH has to be within the normal range at all times. If not, the cells will cease to function properly and a whole lot of serious health problems will develop. If the pH range is not within these values, there could be serious problems. If left untreated, it can turn fatal. However, problems with blood pH only happen as part of disease conditions. The food does not directly affect blood pH.

Thankfully, the body has an effective pH balancing mechanism called the acid-base homeostatic process. This involves the respiratory system and the metabolic system (gut). If the blood pH is acidic, the respirations speed up and the gut slows down to retain more base or alkaline compounds. If the blood pH becomes too alkaline, the respirations slow down and gut movement speeds up to lose more base or alkaline compounds. The urine also plays a part in balancing the blood pH.

What the foods affect is the pH of the urine. This is what the alkaline diet targets.

What makes food alkaline or acidic?

The pH of food in the alkaline diet depends on the pH of the residue once all its components are burned by the body. The most vital rule is that high alkaline foods are those that contain large amounts of alkaline minerals such as potassium, magnesium, sodium and calcium. However, even if a food does contain large amounts of these alkaline minerals, it may still be considered acidic if it also has any of the following:

- Sugar, especially added sugars and refined white sugar

- Fungi, such as mushrooms

- Yeast

- Fermented, such as soy sauce

- Processed, refined or microwaved

These standards explain why it is surprising to see certain acidic foods classified as alkaline in this diet plan. For example, fruits are considered healthy but are classified as acidifying because most of them have high sugar content. The sugar has an acidifying effect in the body. Another example is banana. It is an excellent source of the alkaline mineral potassium. However, it is classified as acidic food because it has about 25% sugar. Other fruits like lemon, lime, avocados and tomatoes are generally thought of as acidic foods, but in the alkaline diet, these fruits are classified as alkaline because these have low sugar.

Sugar is an important determinant in the alkaline diet. The blood can deviate from its normal pH range in the presence of too much sugar. This is a recipe for a double disaster. Too much sugar is a major factor in the development of diabetic condition and all its complications. The excess sugar load in the blood will acidify it and cause even more problems. This is a potent combination that can cause serious chronic health problems such as diabetes and cancer.

The longer this process continues, the more problems arise. These health problems will also become more serious and harder to treat, and all it takes is to simply adjust intake and concentrate on eating more alkaline foods.

What are the Benefits of the Alkaline Diet?

The primary benefit of following the alkaline diet is that it restores or at least brings the body's pH from acidic to more alkaline. Too much acidity can produce lots of health problems and an alkaline diet can help prevent these.

Other benefits of following the alkaline diet go beyond the prevention of symptoms and problems related to too much acid. The alkaline environment helps tissues to function better.

Better energy

Cells must function well in order for the body to produce and use energy well. Acidity interferes with proper cellular processes and reduces energy levels. By going alkaline, the cells can function better. More energy will be produced and the other cells will have more to use for their own functions. This will result to higher energy levels.

Better immunity

When the various cells in the body are healthy, the immune system functions better. The integrity of the cells is great. Cellular integrity protects the cells from infections. The pathogens will find it difficult to enter and cause trouble. If the pH in the body is low (acidic), the cells will find it hard to keep their structures intact. This will allow toxins and pathogens to easily enter and cause more damage. These pathogens and toxins can easily get inside the cells and alter it. This will stimulate the development of health problems. Cancer, for instance, starts off this way. This is also a major reason why some people more frequently get colds and other infections compared to those who follow the alkaline diet.

Reduction in inflammation and pain

Magnesium is an important mineral in the body. It also has a vital role in maintaining the body's pH balance. If the body becomes acidic, the cells will release their magnesium stores to help in neutralizing the acidity. The more acidic the body, the more magnesium is required to counter its effects. This may be ideal but magnesium does not only function for acid neutralizing. The body has so many other uses for magnesium. Using a lot for acid neutralizing can seriously deplete the resources for the other tissues and cellular processes to use.

One of the major tissues affected is the joint. Low magnesium in the body is one of the factors that cause joint diseases and inflammatory conditions. Also, inflammation in the other tissues in the body is also attributed to low magnesium stores. Eating alkaline foods that are also rich in magnesium can replenish the resources and have more for the cells to use.

It strengthens the Neurons

When neurological processes are restored and protected, you get to protect yourself from Alzheimer's

Disease and memory loss. Degenerative diseases could also be prevented.

This happens because alkaline foods also contain L-Theanine, an amino acid that promotes better neurological health—and not a lot of food products are able to do this.

Better Weight Control

This is a culmination of all the positive effects of alkalinity in the body. The cells function better, so that energy is better distributed. Fats are used properly and the body has enough energy. This will reduce cravings and hunger cues. That means reduction in the frequency of hunger cues and better appetite control. Fats and energy are also burned much more efficiently, reducing the risk of accumulating more fats that contribute to weight gain.

Preventing Stomach Upset

Thermogenesis, the term given to fat to energy conversion, is increased by at least 8 to 10 % when someone uses alkaline foods in his daily diet. This not only burns fat, but also regulates the digestive process.

Alkaline foods also reduce intestinal gas, and could also prevent certain diseases from happening, such as ulcers, ulcerative colitis, and Crohn's Disease.

Slower Aging Process

The aging process is driven by the damage to cells. When cells easily degrade and repair is slow, the aging process is accelerated. If the cells are able to repair damage efficiently and at a faster rate, the aging process slows down. In an acidic environment, the cells get easily damaged and at a much faster rate. Repair is slowed in acidic pH. In an alkaline environment, cells do not get as much damage and when any injury gets repaired sooner.

Also, the aging process is accelerated due to oxidative stress. This is caused by the accumulation of free radicals and toxins that eat away at the cells. Acidic pH in the body supports oxidative stress. Alkaline pH helps in reducing the toxin load and oxidative stress. These promote younger-looking, healthier cells that give a younger appearance.

Avoiding Chronic Inflammation

Chronic inflammation is the reason why so many diseases are contracted. These diseases include Type 2 Diabetes, Various Heart Diseases, and Cancer. Many believe this happens because grains are—you guessed it—inflammatory.

Helping to Prevent from Auto-Immune Diseases

Take a look at it this way: Gliadin, also known as the worst kind of gluten, is actually responsible for affecting the pancreas, thyroids, and the entire immune system by means of releasing antibodies that aren't meant to get out yet. When these antibodies go out, auto-immune diseases can be a risk and one may be afflicted with diseases such as Hashimoto's Disease, type 1 diabetes, and hypothyroidism, among others.

Incidentally, research has shown that Alzheimer's Disease is often triggered by high-grain diets. It releasers blockers in the brain that could break mental processes down, and therefore lead to the deterioration of the brain.

Develop a Healthy Gut

Doctors believe that the state of your gut could affect the state of your brain. After all, when you're hungry, you tend to make decisions that are not well thought out.

As you can see, your gut is in charge of a lot of things in your body—which we often fail to see in our daily life. These things include the way you utilize fat and carbohydrates, nutrient absorption, feeling satiated, and vitamin/neurotransmitter production. It can also affect your levels of inflammation, detoxification, and immunity against diseases. (This is not an exhaustive list, these are just some of the factors that stand out).

This is also because of the vagus nerve, found in the gut, which is the longest of the 12 cranial nerves. This is the main channel between your digestive system, and your nerve cells that send signals to the brain.

In short, it's absolutely vital to take gut health seriously since it impacts almost every other facet of our physical health (and one could even argue that it impacts our mental health as well.) Why? Well, because if the given processes above do not work right, you might be afflicted with certain medical conditions, such as dementia, diabetes, allergies, cancer, ADHD, asthma, and other chronic health problems.

Also, when your gut is healthy, your brain gets to make more serotonin—the hormone that keeps you happy and keeps your sanity in check. It's a much better regulator than most anti-depressants.

Avoid Vitamin-D Deficiency

Even if you consume Vitamin D in supplement form, it actually depletes inside the body pretty fast, and acid makes that depletion even faster. Moreover, WGA, or Wheat Germ Agglutinin also causes bacterial growth that kills Vitamin D and damages the gut—and could do much worse to your body in the future.

How to Get Started on the Alkaline Diet

To start the alkaline diet, prepare yourself for a lifetime of dietary changes. It is not a short-term, one-time only diet, even though this is how most people view the term "diet". It is a long-term decision. Knowing the right foods that produce the desired healthy benefits will greatly help you succeed in making your body more alkaline.

Change how you view food

The very first step is to change the way you look at and treat food itself. Take this time to evaluate yourself. Is food merely for sustenance? Is it merely a source of calories? Or is it a source of energy and materials that the body can use to be healthy?

Food should not just be a source of energy. If this is your view, you are likely to be not too concerned on quality. Rather, it's more on quantity. The right thinking should be on the quality of food. The alkaline diet teaches you to be more aware of the things you eat and how they ultimately affect the balance in your body. What are the ingredients in food? Do they supply the body's nutritional requirements? Do they contain potentially harmful components? What is the body's reaction to the various components of food?

Also, never think that diets are just about counting calories. It's important is that you supplement your diet with exercise.

Get a list of the different types of alkaline foods and how they affect the body. A comprehensive list is available at the end of this book. Use this list as a guide on what to include in meals, what to limit and what to avoid.

Drink lots of pure, clean water

Water is vital for normal functioning of the various tissues. In fact, about 70% of the body is composed of water. It is used as a medium for various cellular processes. It is also used to dilute salts, toxins and other substances to keep them under control. Water is used as a medium for excreting wastes and toxins. It is crucial to replenish water stores in the body because it can be easily depleted through sweat, tears, urine, feces, etc.

As the human body is made up of 75% water, it comes as no surprise that a person needs to be able to sustain that amount. If a person loses water in his system, he will be dehydrated and this is dangerous for your physical health. Because of this, it's important to understand how vital water is for you and how much of it you need per day. Water also aids in weight loss. Because it has no preservatives and is not carbonated, it doesn't add any calories or carbohydrates to your body, which is essential for people who want to lose weight.

Surprisingly, water nowadays is acidic. Try to test various commercial bottled water brands and you'll see they are acidic. The usual pH range would be as acidic as pH 4 to 6. Drinking lots of water is good, but not if it's acidic. It will only add more acidity inside the body. Choose clean, pure water. If possible, get spring water, with all the natural dissolved minerals in it. Distilled water in bottles is already stripped off of all the dissolved substances that are beneficial to the body.

Sometimes, the weather gets too hot that a person may feel dehydrated. To prevent being sick or experiencing heat stroke because of extremely hot weather, it's important that a person drinks 13 to 15 cups of water per day or that he eats fruits that are loaded with fluids, too. Aside from water, a person with fever or diarrhea may also have to take oral supplements or sports drinks to replenish the loss of water in his system. You can also try fruits such as watermelons or pears—they're pretty much filled with water and that's why they are good for you.

Also, if you are fond of working out or of any activity that makes you sweat then you certainly need to drink a lot of water to make up for what you have lost. You need to add 1 to 3 more cups to your usual intake.

Aside from water, you could also drink the following:

- **Coconut Water.** Coconut Water is dubbed as nature's own sports drink that has a thermogenic effect and helps make sure that the gut is strong and safe.

- **Juice.** Not the processed kind, though. Try to make your own green juices (with vegetables as base) and mix and match ingredients. It's actually fun, and you'd also help yourself gain a lot of nutrients by doing so, too. Try using the following: *cucumber, celery, beet, carrot, ginger, parsley, spinach, and cabbage.* Then add either of the following: *berries, watermelon, aloe vera, goji berry, acai berry, etc.*

- **Shakes and Smoothies.** Shakes and smoothies are fine, as long as you made them yourself, and they do not contain additives.

- **Tea**. Herbal teas, as you may know by now, are important parts of your diet. Make sure you do not add sugar or milk, though. 3 to 5 cups per day is already good.

The lack of dissolved substances makes distilled water more acidic than regular, clean water. Instead of getting distilled water, choose filtered water. It still retains some of the valuable dissolved materials and is less acidic.

Make various meals out of cruciferous vegetables

Here's the thing: the more alkaline foods you eat, the more weight you'll lose. When you chew alkaline foods, it automatically means that you are already burning and digesting your food—and of course, it's only natural that you get to chew these vegetables, especially if you eat them instead of your usual snacks or fatty foods, in general. If you want to eat your snacks, you need to have the mindset of eating a whole bunch of cruciferous vegetables first—so later, you'd only eat a small amount of the snacks.

Cruciferous vegetables come from the Cruciferae Family. These are vegetables that are generally cultivated for food production. Interestingly, the name also originated from "Cruciferae", which in early Latin literally means "cross-bearing", an allusion to the shape of the flowers that seem to resemble crosses. Prime examples of cruciferous vegetables include: *Brussels sprouts, bok choy, garden cress, broccoli, cabbage,* and *cauliflower.*

These vegetables are known to be essential parts of the Negative Calorie Diet because they are high in cellulose, water, and Vitamin C, together with essential phytochemicals and nutrients that the body needs.

Most cruciferous vegetables also contain glycosylates that are said to prevent cancer, drive toxins away from the body, and could suit the taste of many—and that's why they are used in most plant-based recipes!

You see, your overall calorie intake will ultimately be reduced when you eat alkaline foods instead of high-calorie ones—and if you exercise as you do so, you'd really see substantial amount of weight loss.

Once you start the diet, you'd really notice that you are losing weight. Over time, though, you might feel a lack of energy—but then you'd also realize that as your metabolism slows down, it would then work to provide you with more energy—which will then be used by your body as fuel to live!

What you should keep in mind, though, is that you have to eat at least every 2 to 3 hours—so you can sustain the energy that your body needs, and you also have to take note that you cannot eat sugar or honey—and other sugar replacements, with the exception of Stevia. It's also important not to use any artificial dressings because more often than not, they contain sugar. For dressings, you could use garlic or Dijon mustard mixed with yogurt and your choice of herbs.

How can you make better food choices to improve pH?

Food choices are the cornerstone to improving and balancing pH levels of the body. Everything ultimately depends on what foods were chosen to become part of each and every meal, including snacks. Making the right choice every time is not always easy. To get through the tougher times, live by these guidelines:

- Choose white meat over red meats. Healthier meat alternatives also include meat substitutes and seafood.

- Choose wild rice or yeast-free bread instead of fries or rolls.

- Choose almond milk instead of cow's milk.

- Choose sparkling water instead of alcoholic beverages.

- Choose vegetables as main dishes instead of starches or meats.

- Choose to fill the plate first with plant foods like vegetables, grains and fruits so that there is little space left for acid-forming food items.

- Choose vegetables with dips or fresh grilled fruit instead of prepackaged or processed snacks.

- Choose to use cold-pressed olive oil for cooking instead of butter or saturated fats.

- Choose to have dressings, sauces and condiments on the side instead of having them already mixed into the food when eating out or ordering take-out.

- Choose to exercise every day, like walking for at least 30 minutes instead of watching a 30-minute TV show.

- Choose to reduce the stress levels by performing yoga, meditation and other similar relaxation techniques.

-

How to monitor the pH level of the body?

The simplest and easiest method of monitoring acidity in the body is by checking the urine pH. This is not a requirement to be successful but it helps immensely in checking how well the body responds to the diet. Urine pH monitoring can help in tailoring the diet according to your body's needs. Some people can restore alkalinity by just adding more alkalizing vegetables. Some may need to make huge cut-backs in their meat consumption. Responses are different among individuals and the change is a personal thing. To make the alkaline diet more suitable for your needs, monitor urine pH levels to evaluate your body's responses.

Testing is done every day. Early morning urine is the best sample that can give more reliable results compared to random urine sampling throughout the day. There are ready to use test strips available in pharmacies that you can use to test urine pH levels from the comfort of your home. These test strips can give reliable pH readings without having to take the urine sample to laboratories or medical clinics.

To use the urine pH test strip:

- Remove the test strip from the package. If the test kit comes in a roll, carefully tear off a 3-inch piece.

- Sit down on the toilet bowl and start to urinate. Catch the midstream urine for the test sample. The first few ml of urine (the first 2 seconds worth of urine) is more acidic than the rest and is not the most reliable sample. Readings will give a false positive result. This means getting a very acidic urine pH that's not an actual representation of the entire urine pH. The higher acidity readings is a result of sitting and getting more concentrated in the urinary bladder compared to the rest of the urine.

- Once in midstream, take the urine test strip and place it directly under the stream of urine. Hold it there until the strip is thoroughly moistened.

- Take the test strip then compare it immediately to the chart that comes with the test kit. Match the color of the moistened test strip with the keyed color chart printed on the side of test bottle or of the packaging.

- The number that best matches the color of the test strip will be the urine sample's pH level.

- Record the result. Use this for future reference.

- Discard used test strip properly. These strips are not reusable.

• Testing the urine pH can be done as often as desired. However, once per day is enough to gauge the body's pH level for that day.

The following are the high alkaline foods. Raisins and spinach are among the most alkaline foods.

Alkalizing Vegetables

- Beets

- Broccoli

- Carrots

- Cabbage

- Cauliflower

- Celery

- Collard greens

- Cucumber

- Kale

- Lettuce

- Onion

- Peas

- Pepper

- Spinach

- *Zucchini*

Alkalizing Fruit

- Apples
- Bananas
- Grapes
- Lemon
- Lime
- Melon
- Peach
- Pear
- Orange
- *Watermelon*

Alkalizing Carbohydrates

- Stevia
- Maple syrup
- Rice syrup
- Fresh corn
- Amaranth
- Wild rice
- *Potato skins*

Alkalizing Proteins

- Almonds

- Chestnut

- Goat's milk

- Hazelnuts

- Soybeans

- Tofu

- *Tempeh*

Alkalizing Herbs and Spices

- Basil

- Cinnamon

- Garlic

- Ginger

- Mustard

- *Thyme*

Fats

- Olive oil

- Flaxseed oil

- Canola oil

- *Avocado*

The Acid Alkaline Balance Diet

What is the proper pH balance?

Enzymes or biological molecules within the body are usually proteins, although they may be in other forms. What we eat is broken down by enzymes which act as catalysts in the metabolic processes that sustain our lives. Enzymes cause and speed up chemical reactions in the body which include digestion among other functions.

Enzymes are very selective about which chemical reactions they will speed up. In the body, the way the enzymes behave is affected by the pH level in the body tissues and in the blood. That is why it is essential to maintain the right pH levels for a healthier you. If this is not done, the blood or body tissues may cause diseases which could have otherwise been prevented.

The acid alkaline balance diet is therefore crucial to our health and well-being. You need this diet so that the enzymes can digest the foods properly and promote the absorption of nutrients into the blood to be transported from one part of the body to another.

The acid alkaline balance diet helps the body's metabolism to carry out different functions effectively so that the body eliminates the waste products from the digestive system as it should instead of depositing them in different parts of the body.

The alkaline diet also preserves the sodium, calcium, magnesium and iron in the muscles and bones to prevent them from being offloaded by an alkaline-deficient diet.

This prevents diseases such as arthritis, osteoporosis, multiple sclerosis and lupus. The best alkaline diet promotes health and that is why you should adopt it.

How Acids Affect the Glycemic Index

The Glycemic Index or GI, is basically a guide that tells you how fast carbohydrates get into your bloodstream and turn into sugar, or glucose, which could affect the acidity in your body. There are free online calculators that would help you determine the said amounts but what this chapter will tell you about is how you can manage your GI to make sure that it won't be so high. If you take in a lot of calories, as in more than 1,600, your GI might go higher than usual—so it's best that you take control of that. Basically, what's important is that your body takes a long time to break down carbohydrates into sugar so your body won't be full of sugar and you won't suffer from various ailments. Here are some tips that will help you put your Glycemic Index under control:

1. Know that you can eat as many fruits and vegetables as you like. This is because fruits and vegetables are considered as "Water Foods", which means that they can do no harm to your blood sugar and won't contribute to worsening your situation. However, you have to avoid canned or preserved fruits or vegetables because there are preservatives used in them already and they'll only make your blood sugar levels higher.

2. Eat less-processed or unprocessed grains. No one's asking you to say goodbye to carbohydrates, but you do have to make sure that you eat only the right kinds. This means that you should concentrate on wheat berries, brown rise, millet, and kernel dough instead of rice. Muesli or Granola Breakfast cereals are also fine as long as they are using whole grains and don't contain added sugars and preservatives.

3. Coal foods. Coal foods in particular won't contribute much to your GI because they are high in protein and fiber. Some of the best examples include beans, whole grains, seafood, lean meats, seeds, and nuts, as well as whole-wheat pasta.

4. Avoid fire foods. While coal foods are low in GI, fire foods are very high and that's exactly why you have to avoid them. Some examples include sweet chips, white pasta, white rice, white bread and most heavily processed foods.

5. Stay away from starch. Starchy foods are not good for you because they contribute to your daily GI levels. This means that instead of eating those processed foods or chips for snacks, you should just eat fruits such as pears, papaya, berries, peaches, and apples because they're good for you and they'd add more water to your system.

6. Make sure that you chew your food well and that you eat slowly. When you're eating, you can take as much time as you want because if you chew your food well and if you're not eating in haste, it means that you will be able to avoid having a high Glycemic Index and at the same time, you'd be able to make your metabolic rate go faster, too. When this happens, you get to burn fat quickly and so you also make sure that your health is in tip-top shape.

7. And, find alternatives to the usual foods that you eat. There are days when you seem to crave for foods that aren't really good for you and would just spike up your blood sugar levels. What you can do is find an alternative and eat foods that are in the same category but would still keep your health in check. Check out the list below so you'll have a better idea of what this is about:

- Wild or brown rice instead of white rice.

- Whole wheat instead of regular pasta.

- Rolled or steel-cut oats instead of oatmeal.

- Raisin, oat, muesli, or granola instead of processed corn flakes or breakfast cereals.

- Mashed cauliflower, winter squash, yams, and sweet potatoes instead of mashed or fried white potatoes.

- Leafy greens or peas instead of corn.

- Bran flakes instead of cornflakes.

By following these tips, you can make sure that your Glycemic Index will be in check.

The good news is that there are so many wonderful approaches to maintaining a healthy lifestyle and to losing weight. While some of these diets are more geared towards weight loss others are more geared towards disease prevention and life extension. We've tried to present these diets to you so you can weigh the pros and cons of each one with the desired outcome you hope to achieve and make an educated decision on which approach best suits you (of course after having consulted with your physician).

If you're all about the support and you want someone to make all the decisions for you and do all the facts and figuring, Weight Watchers might be your ideal choice. If you want to be able to eat whatever you want and don't mind adhering to a very strict eating schedule, Intermittent Fasting might make all the difference for you. If you're seeking to make a life change and detoxify your body the Alkaline Diet might be worth the effort.

Whatever you decide, remember that your effort and commitment are more important than choosing the right diet. Measure and track your success, drawn on support options available to you, stay in consultation with your doctor, and do your utmost to stay committed and cut out whatever is keeping you from success. Periodically re-evaluate and make adjustments as needed. Remember your diet is supposed to work for you (not the other way around).

Your options have been laid before you but your success depends on you.

9 781724 618986